Alive &

Kicking

The Carer's Guide to Exercises for Older People

Julie Sobczak

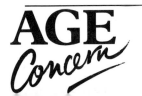

AGE Concern

BOOKS

Coventry University

© 2001 Julie Sobczak

Published by Age Concern England
1268 London Road
London SW16 4ER

First published 2001

Editor Richenda Milton-Thompson
Production Vinnette Marshall
Designed and typeset by GreenGate Publishing Services, Tonbridge, Kent
Printed and bound in Great Britain by Bell & Bain Ltd, Glasgow
Photographs by Jon Stewart

A catalogue record for this book is available from the British Library

ISBN 0-86242-289-2

Bulk orders
Age Concern England is pleased to offer customised editions of all its titles to UK
companies, institutions or other organisations wishing to make a bulk purchase.
For further information, please contact the Publishing Department at the address
on this page. Tel: 020 8765 7200. Fax: 020 8765 7211. Email: books@ace.org.uk

Contents

About the author and contributors

The author

Julie Sobczak, BSc (Hons), Dip.N, RM, RN, YMCA, RSA has been a nurse for over 25 years here in the UK and in the West Indies. She has also been developing exercise classes for all age groups in the Yorkshire area over the last ten years, specialising in exercises for older people since 1992. In addition, Julie is a regular contributor to nursing journals in the field of health and exercise.

Contributors

Susie Dinan is the Senior Clinical Exercise Practitioner and a Research Fellow in the Department of Primary Care and Population Sciences, Old Age Psychiatry and Health Services for Elderly People at the Royal Free and University College School of Medicine.

Piers Simey is Physical Activity Adviser for Merton, Sutton and Wandsworth Health Authority.

*F*oreword

With an increasingly ageing population, the burden of disability is likely to increase. As a society, our objectives should be to prevent and postpone illness and morbidity and to improve healthy, active life expectancy. With early intervention, correct diagnosis, treatment and rehabilitation, the most important single sequel to any illness in old age – disability – can be avoided. Similarly, with positive and active health measures and changes in lifestyle, the quality of life can be significantly improved and, in many instances, illnesses and subsequent disabilities can also be prevented. In that sense, 'prevention' is the most cost-effective health policy.

Physical activity and regular exercise for older people is being encouraged as a very effective, preventive health measure. Julie Sobczak's work on 'active living' is therefore, timely and most welcome. In this book, she has presented strong arguments in favour of remaining physically active and effective in the later years of life in an easily digestible way. She has given very sensible advice and her instructions on exercise procedures are practical and easy to follow.

I would strongly recommend this book, not only to health professionals and health promotion experts but to all individuals from middle age onwards, so that they can 'get into the swing of things' and allow quality life to enrich their later years.

Dr Arup K. Banerjee OBE, JP, FRCP (Lond., Edin.,Glas., Irel.)
Director of Elderly Services
South Manchester University Hospitals NHS Trust
Immediate Past President, British Geriatrics Society

*A*cknowledgements

Thank you to the residents and staff of Anley Hall, Gargrave Park, Stainforth House and Milton House – all in North Yorkshire, for the years of fun we've had together in our quest to keep fit; to Susie Dinan for arranging the photo shoot and contributing the very important chapter on Safety; to Piers Simey for his equally important contribution from a Health Promotion Perspective; to all the models who so generously gave their time and energy for the photographs which help to explain the exercises – May Allen, Bill Badger, Sybil Bowen, Ben Eley, Ellen Glover Lewis, Pat Howard, Vivien Milroy, Irene Nahon and Victor Rosen; to my husband Vic for his patience and love; to my father in law Joe who included exercise into his daily routine until his death in 2000 at the age of 91; to my mother in law Chrissy who also recognises the value of exercise despite numerous recent illnesses and difficulties; and to everyone at Age Concern, especially Richard Holloway; to Marks and Spencer for sponsoring most of the models' clothing and Jon Stewart for taking the photographs. This project would not have been possible without the generous support and contributions of all these people.

Introduction

The adult population is the largest it has ever been in the history of the United Kingdom, and it is still growing. Since 1951 the percentage of the UK population over the age of 65 has more than doubled. It is the 85+ age group that is increasing fastest, with for example, a 200 per cent increase in growth projected for centenarians during the first three decades of the 21st Century[1] Buckingham Palace confirm that congratulatory telemessages from The Queen sent to new centenarians has increased tenfold since 1955. Additionally, 389 people in 1998 received telegrams for their 105th birthday, or over[2].

Many of us see ageing as something just to dread. Certainly popular culture holds many negative stereotypes of what it means to be old. We may fear losing our independence, family and homes as illness, frailty and infirmity mean that these end years must be spent in care. An ageing society, with a growing number becoming more dependent on health and social services, makes maintaining health and postponing chronic disease a high priority.

In most western cultures, old age and illness are often seen as the same thing. However, studies have shown that ageing, inactivity and illness are different from each other, although these factors together can cause or promote premature mental and physical disability. Regular, simple exercises in a context of healthy eating and living can help to maintain our ability to function on our own. Research into ageing and exercise has shown that exercise can increase the stamina of an older person and increase the capacity for independent living by as much as 10–20 years[3].

Even those people who require residential or nursing home care can live a more active and independent life if they are given help and support to do this. I recall my early experiences caring for those in residential and nursing homes. Busy, often understaffed homes had inflexible regimes for residents who spent endless hours just sitting staring blankly at each other or at a television screen. Only meal times and 'toileting' punctuated their long and empty days. If residents were not confused and depressed when they came to the home, it was clear that many of them became so when mental and physical stimulation was such a low priority or even considered 'unnecessary'. These circumstances often defined their final identity, smothering past identities based upon previous lives which included family, work, activities and interests. Thank goodness this dismal picture is changing. Nursing and residential homes are slowly embracing rehabilitation into their philosophy of care as evidence grows that regular activity throughout the day increases the probability of a higher quality of life.

There are many exercise programmes and information available for younger people to enhance quality of life. But this is generally not the case for those aged 75 or over, even though the benefits can be considerable.

This book looks at the role of exercise for older people and offers instruction in the kind of exercises that are suitable for this often forgotten group. I give particular attention to those older people who may be in care and therefore require the assistance of others for support with daily living activities and safe exercise programmes. If you are a health professional, nursing or residential home manager, activity organiser, relative or carer involved with older people, you will find this book useful for developing a body of knowledge about appropriate movements to enhance older peoples' lives.

The promotion of physical activity is the responsibility of many agencies but we, as health professionals and carers involved in the day to day care of older people, can recognise our unique opportunity to influence older peoples' lives in a positive manner. The evidence is hard to ignore; people who exercise regularly are more likely to maintain bone and muscle mass, stamina, power and suppleness. Important additional mental benefits include improved social confidence, mood and self-esteem.[4] A fun, lively activity session also adds variety to the day and promotes camaraderie. When the ability to function on our own is maintained or improved we can look forward to a more dignified end.

There are now courses available for those who wish to go further and qualify as exercise teachers for older adults. Details of these courses can be found in Chapter 4 and the Resources section of this book. Such a course will teach you essential basic principles of exercise physiology and how to apply these so you can conduct safe and successful activity sessions with older people. For a variety of reasons, however, it may not be possible for everyone interested in learning more about exercise to take a formal exercise teaching course, although this is strongly recommended where possible. Safe practice is of course of paramount consideration, but the absence of specific training need not prevent you from helping older people to become more active. This book will give carers and older people themselves the knowledge necessary to become involved in enjoyable and meaningful exercises. The exercises described are largely mild chair based movements that are selected for their potential to maintain or increase range of motion, stamina, flexibility and strength.

In addition to improving the quality of life for older adults you may discover a welcome side effect for nursing staff and carers as older people assume more control over their mobility and self care activities. Mood improves dramatically when people feel they have regained even the smallest amount of control over their lives. This in turn leads to a more positive, happier environment for everyone. So go for it! As Dr Arup Banerjee (past President of the British Geriatrics Society) suggests, we should aim not to just keep everyone alive but rather we should aim to help keep people 'alive and kicking'[5].

■ Research into ageing and exercise has shown that exercise can increase the stamina of an older person and extend the capacity for independent living by as much as 10–20 years.

Source: Aoyagi & Shephard[3]

Benefits of chair work

Chair work has the following benefits. It:

- Stabilises the lumbar spine by providing a fixed base. This particularly assists those people with lordosis, kyphosis and other postural problems, to mobilise the spine as effectively as possible.
- Facilitates teaching of correct technique, especially for more complex exercises (eg trunk twists).
- Facilitates greater range of movement (ROM) by providing points of leverage and support, eg utilising the chairback in trunk twists achieves a larger range than is possible without a chair.
- Encourages controlled performance by returning to the centre each time and by restricting trunk movements.
- Facilitates training of functional capacity by providing a solid base of support.

- Provides upper and lower body stretches and mobility work, eg hamstring and triceps stretches, quadriceps and abductor strengthening, ankle mobility work.
- Minimises load-bearing, reduces balance problems and, therefore, increases comfort and confidence.
- Facilitates a mix of exercise intensity and type (endurance and resistance, balance) that would be impossible for less able individuals in free-standing positions.
- Facilitates the link with life situations, eg sit and stand, triceps press, lifting technique, getting up and down from the floor or bed.
- Facilitates social interaction because, whether in a circle, circuit, line or partner formation, chair work tends to stimulate chatting.

References

1 *Research into Ageing: Annual Report* (1996/97). Baird House, London.

2 Personal Communication with Mr David Tuck, Assistant Press Secretary to the Queen (1999). Buckingham Palace, London.

3 Aoyagi, Y. and Shephard, R.J. (1992) Ageing and Muscle Function. *Sports Medicine*, Issue 6, Vol.14, December 1992 p376–396. Auckland.

4 Norman, K.A. (1995) Exercise programming for older adults. *Human Kinetics*, Montana State University.

5 A Banerjee (1998) Meeting expectations. *Research into Ageing News*, Issue 10 (Winter).

Chapter 1

What is fitness?

Early definitions of health considered fitness as merely the absence of disease. In 1959 the World Health Organisation extended this definition to include a sense of 'fitness' rather than just the absence of disease or infirmity. You are almost certain to have your own ideas about what fitness means. Perhaps it ranges from being able to climb a flight of stairs without getting exhausted to being able to complete or even win a marathon. Fitness to me means being able to do my work and still have some energy left at the end of the day. I also need to be fit to swim, walk and play squash without getting breathless and exhausted. These are also the activities I do in order to keep fit. When I feel fit, I feel healthy – although fitness and health do not always go together. We have all heard of those athletes and sports people (for example, ballet dancers and racing jockeys) who have starved their bodies in order to keep weight down.

What does fitness mean to older people?

In particular, what does being fit mean to those who live in residential or nursing homes? Through informal interviews with residents of nursing homes I discovered that their definitions were many, but that everyone valued and wanted to achieve a 'functional' fitness. For example, being able to accomplish a particular task such as dressing without assistance. No-one wanted to play squash or run a marathon, but they wanted to be able to 'get about' as much as possible and 'not have to rely on others too much'.

Set up your own discussion group with older people, friends and colleagues. It is a useful way to build rapport and understand other people's view of fitness in relation to their changing needs and circumstances. And it's good fun! Indeed, the success of any activity programme is greatly increased if it includes ideas from participants. Such a discussion group helps you and your colleagues to examine your own personal ideas of health and fitness along with those in your care. I would like to share just a few comments from two nursing home residents I spoke with – Mrs J and Mrs P are both in their late eighties.

Mrs J: I used to walk a lot myself but I've had a lot of falls just recently and I can't do it now.

Mrs P: I still enjoy my walking.

Mrs J: Oh I used to enjoy it. When I went to the hospital after I broke my wrist they sent me to the rehabilitation unit and they asked me if I wanted to continue with the classes so I said yes. They came for me (to my home) in the morning and brought me back in the afternoon and we had our lunch there and we met other people and it was nice to talk to other people … I think if someone could come to do exercises … and encourage people to try those other exercises.

Mrs P: It isn't a worry for me because I know I can still walk, but I know it must be a worry for other people.

Mrs J: It is a worry. When I used to do the exercises with the physiotherapist I got to so that I could walk – not without help of course, but I wasn't doing so badly. Now it's all gone you see. They just seem to cut you off … and we don't get anything like that anymore. I asked if I could go from here but they said they haven't the staff to take me. I'm sure a lot of people would have kept going if they had encouragement.

They just seem to cut you off … just to dump you somewhere and do nothing after you've had these exercises and be left with no-one bothering whether you carry on or not … it isn't right is it?

Who is old?

Most of us will experience old age – if we live long enough! Yet old age is still a subject that is misunderstood or even avoided. It is not surprising that many of the older people I meet tell me that the old days were the best times. These were the times they felt most useful, active and wanted.

We still talk about 'geriatrics' or 'pensioners' as if older people become part of an homogenised lump at retirement age, with no future, dreams or goals. Our society offers few opportunities for older people to contribute in a positive and productive way. Families move away from each other and contact with the generations is lost or sporadic. No wonder many younger people hold grim visions of ageing and find it difficult to imagine older people as having anything to offer this fast changing world.

'Old age'

Retirement age may be a useful bureaucratic marker, but it fails to help us understand the real meaning of 'old age'. What matters most is not how old a person is (ie the calendar age), but their functional (or biological) age. There is no standard, typical, or even average older person. Old age covers a wide range of individuals, male and female, whose previous experiences may have included roles and occupations such as farming, armed services, teaching, law, parenting, medicine and nursing. Indeed, the only common thread connecting 'old people' is that they are unique individuals who are ever changing according to time, health and environmental circumstances.

We all know younger people who appear to be 'old before their time' and others, such as Kathleen, my neighbour who delivers the daily papers around the village and who has a spirit and vigour that belies her 81 years. Kathleen was awarded the MBE in 1993 for her lifetime service to others. Kathleen tells me that her wish to remain as independent as possible will remain her focus so that she can continue to help others.

Independence

The wish for independent living is a common aim for older people no matter if they live in their own homes, sheltered housing or in residential and nursing homes. Retaining autonomy means more than being able to stay in one's home. However, when people are faced with health problems there may be an increased feeling of dependency and loss of autonomy. Social networks are broken, confidence, self-esteem and self-worth may also be eroded, leading sometimes to depression and mental illness. Loss of family and friends and a fear for the future only serve to compound these problems.

Surprisingly, however, many older people have to go into care, not because of ill health, disease or mental impairment, but simply because of muscle weakness. Once in a care home, if activity is not built into the normal day, muscle weakness will continue to increase, resulting in a further deterioration of fitness. This is often the scenario in care homes where rehabilitation is not genuinely addressed.

Choice and autonomy

Most of us are fortunate enough to have the choice to exercise or not, and if we choose to be active there are a variety of activities, clubs, organisations, equipment and suitably trained people to meet our needs. Many older people however are not so fortunate and go into care because they are unable to meet their own needs. They may dread this move as it often means giving up their own home, but worst of all, they fear their autonomy will be sacrificed. Moving into a care home should not mean losing choices or being totally disconnected from the life they once knew. Although there have often been negative associations attached to institutionalised care, the mood is changing as managers and health workers in care homes work hard to fulfil philosophies that safeguard residents' independence.

Abigail chose to move to a nursing home in her late eighties when her eyesight and hearing seriously deteriorated. This change was seen as a positive move by Abigail who says she feels more secure in a place where there is expert help should she need it. Although quite frail, she is mentally fit and able to walk very slowly with the aid of walking sticks. Abigail has always been very active and tells me that she misses being busy in her own home. She attends most of the exercise sessions offered at the home because she says they 'help to keep the joints from seizing up'.

Another resident told me she is 'past it' for exercising. Florence, who is also in her late eighties, has lived in care for several years. Her mobility is quite poor and she has dementia problems, but she manages to walk short distances with the aid of a zimmer frame. I never fail to invite Florence to the exercise sessions and she regularly turns down these invitations, preferring to remain in her favourite chair in the reception area. Yet once the familiar music starts, Florence begins to take an interest in the exercise group. Soon after, Florence can be seen slowly heading towards the class, scanning the room for a spare seat. So now there is always a vacant seat quite near the door, made available just for Florence. Others tell me they would like to just sit and listen to the music, and they are certainly welcome to do this. Yet rarely are they able to just sit and watch, toes start tapping, some clap their hands and join in with the sing-a-long tunes that are often just too tempting to ignore.

Finally, I cannot resist mentioning the French lady Madame Calment who, until her recent death, was the oldest person in the world at 122 years. Madame Calment claimed to have reached this age because she laughed a lot and exercised regularly. She took up fencing at the age of 85, cycled up until she was 100 and did not enter a nursing home until the age of 110.

The value of exercise

Until recently, older people were rarely included in studies researching the health benefits of regular physical activity. In 1992 a Government report, *The Health of the Nation*[1], recognised that physical activity or exercise is as fundamental to healthy living, as food and sleep. The report further emphasised the role of activity as a means to preserve independence in older people and those with a disability.

Fitness survey

In 1992 a major study, *The Allied Dunbar National Fitness Survey*[2], investigated the physical activity levels of the British population. It discovered a high proportion of people over 55 years of age were failing to carry out the tasks of daily living because of inadequate strength; 40 per cent of those in the 65–74 year old group took no vigorous or moderate exercise. Meanwhile, 30 per cent of men and 50 per cent of women aged 65–74 did not have sufficient strength in their thigh muscles to power their legs efficiently. If this is the position for so many people approaching the age of 75, then what about the years after the age of 75? The report did hold some good news, however. It found that, despite the ageing process, exercise can play a major part in reversing these low performance trends. This means we can no longer accept the idea that a progressive loss of function and general decline is simply a consequence of ageing.

Common health problems

Although there are several factors that contribute to a healthy, independent old age (such as environment, finance, nutrition and access to medical care), activity can play a major part in helping older people to remain agile and independent throughout their remaining years. Regular exercise can optimize levels of fitness required for the daily tasks of living, encourage social contacts, improve the general feeling of wellbeing, maintain muscle tissue, increase appetite and help to avoid day to day problems such as constipation[3]. It might be useful at this stage to look at some of these common health problems and the potential value of exercise in these circumstances.

Leg ulcers

These are often due to poor circulation, weakened, damaged and narrowed blood vessels. Walking and exercises that mimic a walking action play an important role in activating the calf muscle pump. During such exercise the calf muscle contracts and relaxes against the veins. This acts as a pump to force the blood up the leg and towards the heart. This movement can be quite difficult if the ankle is stiff and immobile, so the exercise must be tailored to the ability and flexibility of the individual. Exercise must be postponed in legs that are painful and inflamed.

Gravitational oedema

This commonly occurs when the circulation becomes stagnated. Fluid from the circulatory system leaks into the tissue, gravity encourages this leakage to find the lowest level, which is the lower legs and ankles when sitting in a chair. Inactivity makes this condition much worse. Walking and/or ankle exercises can help to reduce swelling, combined with periods of rest with the feet raised.

Pressure sores

A pressure sore is an area where the skin and tissues have been damaged because of inactivity and prolonged contact with a hard surface. They can affect just the skin or be so deep that they reach the bone. Pressure sores are also known as bed sores. The most common areas to be affected include the sacrum, shoulder blades, heels, elbows, and the back of the head. Frail older people with mobility problems are especially vulnerable as they are often unable to change position or even shuffle around in the bed or chair. Movement is crucial for the prevention of pressure sores. Strengthening exercises are also vital for individuals to be able to maintain or develop sufficient power to be able to lift their own weight (from a chair) and so relieve pressure areas.

Constipation

Constipation is quite common in older people, particularly if the diet lacks roughage (fibre) and there is inadequate fluid intake to help the waste to pass easily along the colon. Activity is also playing an increasing role in the prevention of constipation. Those who include some form of activity in their daily lives experience fewer problems with colon function.

Sleep

Poor quality sleep can be linked to a variety of factors. Many older people describe feelings of anxiety and agitation before bedtime and report problems with sleeplessness. Sleep disruption has been shown to exaggerate medical conditions and erode quality of life. Even when we are in the best of health, sleep problems can leave us feeling tense, irritable and unable to cope. If sleep is necessary for recuperation and restoration, it is easy to see how those who are sleep deprived may suffer from memory deficits, fatigue and personality changes. Whilst activity late in the day can produce over stimulation and add to difficulties in sleeping, a little light exercise during the day may help to prepare for a more efficient quality of sleep by inducing feelings of tiredness and well being. Chapter 8 talks a little more about sleep and how relaxation exercises can help to get rid of tension and stress.

Nutrition

Many older people have a lowered appetite for food which may lead to an inadequate daily intake of essential nutrients. Introducing activity may help to boost appetite and so increase the intake of vitamins, minerals and calories to decrease these risks.

Mind and mood

There are claims that physical fitness can jog the memory and stimulate the mind, possibly as a result of an increased oxygen supply to the brain whilst exercising[4]. There have also been improvements reported in those who suffer from negative emotional states. Some of the older people I work with suffer from depression and anxiety resulting from sudden changes in their lives. For example, Ingrid lived in her own home and was completely self caring until a sudden, severe stroke robbed her of her independence. Ingrid clearly held a negative attitude towards her disabilities and she was often angry or depressed. Following her stroke, Ingrid was transferred to a residential home after a short stay in hospital, never returning to the home in which she had spent her whole adult life. Initially, Ingrid 'couldn't see the point' of exercise for someone like herself, but agreed to 'have a go'. Ingrid has now started to mix with the other residents, and there is an increased optimism and spirit in her manner. Instead of constantly talking about the things she can't do, she is now finding out about the things she can do.

Dementia

Those suffering from dementia problems may have low activity levels even when there is no physical disability. Altered brain function may interfere with a person's ability to maintain confidence, balance and perception when mobile, thus increasing vulnerability to falls, isolation and depression. Many of the participants in my movement classes have mental health problems including dementia, Parkinson's disease and Alzheimer's disease. Although communication can be difficult, I find many of those with mental impairment can follow simple instructions or mimic some of the moves. Even low levels of activity may have vital benefits that can help to minimise the effects of disability and disease, create opportunities for socialisation and postpone or reduce further depression and dependence[5].

Stroke

The period of inactivity following a stroke will further compromise a person's level of fitness and independence. Slow, controlled moves that follow the range of motion can help to prevent joint contracture and the wasting away of muscles that can still function[6]. Never move a person's limbs or joints for them, only a qualified therapist can do this safely.

Arthritis

One of the major causes of arthritis has been attributed to ageing. Yet in one study of older people (70–79 year olds) a significant percentage of older people (15 per cent) remained free of arthritic changes in their joints[7]. Results from other studies suggest it is a lack of normal movement which causes joint stiffness and cell changes in the cartilage. These changes may in turn lead to arthritis. Exercise, especially full range and weight bearing movement, plays a major role in joint nutrition and preservation[7]. However, exercise is not recommended for the older person with injured or painful joints[7].

Loneliness

Exercise sessions are a great way of getting people together. Loneliness and withdrawal from society can occur in older people even when they are in a busy residential home. Loneliness can be as a result of recent bereavement, loss of contact with friends and relatives, failing health and disability. This can lead to apathy, boredom, loss of self esteem and self neglect. Exercise can definitely play a role in increasing social interaction. Earlier I mentioned Ingrid who was initially reluctant to join the activity classes. Something rather wonderful happened when she attended one of the activity classes. Ingrid recognised a new lady in the class who had come to the home for respite care. They discovered they had been to the same school together – over 70 years ago! Ingrid said she would never have met her friend if she had remained alone in her room. Of course there is always the risk that classes can become more of a social meeting than a way to improve physical fitness. One way to strike the correct balance is by providing plenty of opportunity following the activity part of the class for general discussion and friendly chat.

- Chronic illness or physical injury does not necessarily prevent a person from exercising
- Most chronic conditions improve with proper exercise

Source: Fiatarone et al.[8]

References

1 Department of Health (1992) *The Health of the Nation.* HMSO, London.

2 Health Education Authority and the Sports Council. (1992) *Allied Dunbar National Fitness Survey: Main Findings. Report on Activity Patterns and Fitness Levels.* Belmont Press, Northampton.

3 Fentem, P.H. (1994) Benefits of exercise in health and disease. *British Medical Journal,* Vol 308 (14th May) pp.1291–1295.

4 Martini, F. (1992) *Fundamentals of Anatomy and Physiology.* Prentice Hall, New Jersey: pp. 471–497.

5 Dinan, S. (1998) Fit for life: Why exercise is vital for everyone. *Journal of Dementia Care,* Vol 6, No 3, pp.22–25.

6 Spirduso, W.W. (1995) *Physical dimensions of ageing.* Human Kinetics. Champagne, Illinois.

7 Norris, C. (1999) Body mechanics: joints and ageing. *Exercise (Publication of the National Governing Body for Exercise & Fitness in England).* Jan/Feb, p.15.

8 Fiatarone, M.A, O'Brien K., Brent S.E.RKH, MD (1996) Exercise Rx for a healthier old age. *Patient Care,* October 15, pp. 145–158.

Chapter 2

*H*ow our bodies change in old age

'If I knew I was going to live this long I would have taken better care of myself.'

Eubie Blake – age 100

Few of us think seriously about what kind of older person we might become. Perhaps we think it is better to cross that bridge when we come to it. It is an accepted fact that degenerative changes are inevitable with increased age. Yet this ageing process affects us all at different rates. Why do some individuals maintain a functional level of health and fitness well into old age? Can age-related changes be slowed down or prevented by changes in lifestyle? As exercise leaders we need to understand how the ageing process affects our body systems and how these systems can be enhanced by safe and appropriate exercise.

Musculoskeletal fitness

Joints, tendons and ligaments

The skeletal system includes bones, joints, tendons and ligaments. Movement occurs when the skeletal system interacts with the muscular system[1]. The strength and flexibility of tendons and ligaments are essential for joint stability and full range of movement.

Effects of ageing

Ageing reduces the strength and stability in the joints, tendons and ligaments. A loss of strength in these translates into less body control which in turn leads to joint injury, muscle strains or tendon and ligament damage. There is no point having strong bones if these supporting structures are weak and stiff.

Exercise benefits

Careful stretching and exercises which provide resistance can promote suppleness in the muscles, tendons and ligaments. Exercise also helps to prevent the loss of muscle tissue which is important for strength, and good body control[1].

Bones

The bones of the skeleton are living tissue, constantly undergoing renewal by the process of 're-modelling'. In younger people old bone is absorbed and new bone is laid down at about the same rate so that bone mass is retained.

Effects of ageing[2]

As we age, old bone is absorbed at a faster rate than new bone can be formed. This results in bones becoming less dense, brittle (osteoporosis) and highly vulnerable to injury and fracture. Other factors influencing bone loss include poor nutrition, smoking, alcohol intake and the onset of menopause in women. A further major cause of bone loss is when there is a lack of stress (inactivity) on the bones. This was dramatically observed in astronauts on their return from the weightless environment of space. These days, when astronauts take to space they follow a programme of daily exercise to limit bone loss.

Exercise benefits[2]

Current studies show that physical activity and weight bearing exercises can maintain or improve bone density. Weight bearing exercise refers to activities where the body is moved from one place to another – for example, walking, stair climbing or dancing. Those older people who are unable to participate in weight bearing activities can improve or maintain bone mass with resistance training which means using their muscles to lift (or resist) weights. In resistance training the muscle also becomes stronger and larger in response to lifting or resisting increasing loads.

Even those who doubt the influence of exercise on bone density say exercise is vital be because it improves physical balance and co-ordination which may help reduce the risk of injury from falling. This in itself is a major consideration since the consequences of a fall are very serious and a major source of hospital and nursing home admissions[3] (see Table 2.1).

Table 2.1 The costs of falls

- An older person who falls is more likely to fall again
- The risk of falling increases dramatically with age
- 50 per cent of those who live in residential homes fall at least once a year
- Fractures resulting from falls cost the NHS about £750 million each year

Although minor falls may not result in fractures, they may cause

- loss of confidence
- reduced mobility
- the need for extra care and support

Source: Skelton[4]

Muscle strength

We would not be able to move without our muscles. They provide the pulling power that make our bones move, give shape to the bony skeleton and generate heat to keep us warm. Muscle strength and muscle power (how fast you can exert your strength) is necessary throughout life in order to function well in work, family life and leisure pursuits. Preserving muscle tissue becomes even more important in old age as loss of muscle strength in an already frail older person may mean there is no longer adequate strength for safe walking or independent living. In such cases, muscle power may have deteriorated to a level where the individual is unable to lift his or her own weight to move from chair to toilet seat or from chair to bed.

Effects of ageing

Although muscle mass (or muscle size) deteriorates as a consequence of old age, there is increasing evidence to show that it is inactivity rather than merely 'old age' which induces the greatest reported rate of muscle loss[2].

Exercise benefits

The good news is that older people can benefit by strength training[2]. There has been a great deal of success with strength training programmes aimed at building leg strength in frail older people. One such programme in Boston (USA) produced spectacular changes in a small group of care home residents whose average age was 90 years old. The individuals in the study shared the same kind of problems that might be seen in any care home, such as multiple chronic diseases, functional disabilities, and a history of long term sedentary habits. Results from the study showed an average increase in strength of 174 per cent. Some of the participants actually experienced a three or fourfold increase in strength. More importantly, these results translated into practical functional abilities such as improved walking. Just as spectacular was the speedy decline of muscle strength in these individuals once the training study ended. The group showed a 32 per cent loss in muscle strength in just three weeks after the training study was stopped[5].

A recent British study[6] of men and women aged 80–93 showed that women increased their aerobic power (increased stamina to perform the same or similar activities for longer periods) by 15 per cent after 24 weeks (three exercise sessions a week) of endurance training. The study also showed that women over 80 could improve their stamina as much as younger women in training – but that these improvements in older women would take longer to achieve. The men in the study however showed no improvements and this is thought to be because their starting level of fitness was much higher. So once again we have evidence that it is never too late to improve or maintain a level of fitness which supports a higher quality of life as we age.

Fitness and other body systems

The circulatory system

The circulatory system includes the heart, lungs and blood vessels. This system transports blood around the body to remove waste products and supply tissues with oxygen and nourishment.

Effects of ageing

With age the blood vessels lose elasticity and become rigid (a condition commonly known as hardening of the arteries). There may also be some degree of narrowing or obstruction in the vessels. Blood pressure is raised as the heart works harder to pump the blood through these damaged blood vessels which in turn contributes to heart enlargement and disease[7].

The lungs and its supporting structures (muscles, blood vessels and rib cage) also lose elasticity. There are fewer air sacs (alveoli) in the lungs resulting in reduced air exchange. This means that breathing becomes more difficult and less efficient. These changes may cause the individual to become tired and breathless very quickly.

Exercise benefits

The heart is a muscular pump, capable of responding to exercise like other muscles in the body. A lifetime of endurance activities and sports can help to keep this system strong and capable of coping with daily living tasks and sudden bursts of activity such as sprinting for a bus. Such a lifestyle also sows the seeds for an active and independent old age. Conversely, individuals who have led a mostly sedentary life are most likely to suffer from the debilitating effects of disuse.

Endurance is when we have sufficient power to repeatedly perform an exercise or activity. Increasing activities strengthen the heart and lungs. Circulation may also be improved as blood is efficiently pumped around the body in order to supply enough oxygen to the working muscles.

Even minor physical improvements can have positive effects on functioning. For example Annie, who attends weekly art therapy classes in addition to exercise classes in her residential home told me, 'I can paint for longer now without falling asleep'. Annie is sedentary for most of the day, in an armchair or for short periods in a wheelchair. She is very tiny and frail-looking and depends on her carers for everyday activities. Yet Annie, at 96 years of age, is one of my most enthusiastic class participants and can maintain simple leg and arm (sometimes both together) exercises for increasingly lengthy periods.

An exercise regime for this particular group of older people obviously needs to be chosen carefully. Warning symptoms such as shortness of breath, chest pain, sweating, and undue fatigue must be closely monitored. Problems can be avoided if activity is tailored to each person's physical and medical condition. For example, I notice Mary gets quite breathless as she moves around the sitting room. However, she is keen to join in with the chair exercise sessions and manages to follow the simple, slow moves without problems. Mary is closely observed for signs of distress and encouraged to keep her arms low so her heart does not have to work as hard. This level of activity can be increased slowly as Mary adapts to each new change.

The nervous system

The nervous system acts as the computer responsible for the co-ordinated activity of the whole body. This system is busy 24 hours a day sending and receiving messages between the brain, spinal cord and nerve endings. The quality of our lives is determined by our nervous system which allows us to control the way our bodies move, gives us consciousness and shapes our individual personalities[8].

Effects of ageing

By the age of 30 the ageing process has started to affect the nervous system. Nerve cells progressively die and are not replaced. There is some loss of short term memory and a slowing of reaction and movement time. In addition, hearing, smell and vision may also become less acute. When balance, co-ordination, speed and movement control is affected this may interfere with ability to function safely and effectively. In practical terms, this may mean difficulty in accomplishing everyday tasks, and even more seriously, increase the risks of stumbling or falling.

Exercise benefits

Once again, debate continues on exactly how much deterioration of the nervous system is due to the ageing process alone. Nevertheless there is evidence to show that, regardless of age, those groups who are physically active have much faster reaction times than corresponding age groups that are less active[8].

In conclusion, irrespective of whether a decline in function is the result of ageing or inactivity, it is clear that inactivity can promote and accelerate some of the debilitating effects often associated with old age (see Figure 2.1). Exercise may not necessarily provide the complete answer to a healthy old age free of disabilities, but increasing research into this area shows it can play a major role in interrupting the vicious cycle of immobility and dependence[9].

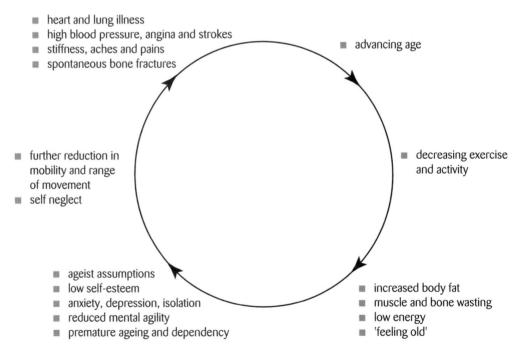

■ heart and lung illness
■ high blood pressure, angina and strokes
■ stiffness, aches and pains
■ spontaneous bone fractures

■ advancing age

■ further reduction in mobility and range of movement
■ self neglect

■ decreasing exercise and activity

■ ageist assumptions
■ low self-esteem
■ anxiety, depression, isolation
■ reduced mental agility
■ premature ageing and dependency

■ increased body fat
■ muscle and bone wasting
■ low energy
■ 'feeling old'

Figure 2.1. The Exercise–Ageing Cycle
Adapted from The Academy Papers: Spirduso & Eckert[10]

References

1 Norman, K.A. (1995) Exercise programming for older adults. *Human Kinetics*. Champagne, Illinois.

2 Spirduso, W.W. (1995) Physical dimensions of ageing. *Human Kinetics*. Champagne, Illinois.

3 Tibbits, G.M. (1996) Patients who fall: how to predict and prevent injuries. *Geriatrics*, Vol.51, No. 9 (Sept.) p.24.

4 Skelton, D. (1998) Prevention of falls. *Research into Ageing News*. Issue 9 (Sept.).

5 Fiatarone, M.A., Marks E.C., Ryan, N.D. *et al.* (1990) High intensity strength training in nonagenarians: Effects on skeletal muscle. *Journal of the American Medical Association*, 26, pp.3029–3034.

6 *Research into Ageing News* (1998) Can the 80+ age group increase their physical fitness? Issue 10 (winter).

7 Laing, W. and Hall, M. (1991) *Demographic Trends – Agenda for Health: The Challenges of Ageing.*, Association of the British Pharmaceutical Industry, London.

8 Martini, F. (1992) *Fundamentals of Anatomy and Physiology*. Prentice Hall, New Jersey, pp. 471–497.

9 Krucoff, C. (1994) Use 'em or lose 'em. *Saturday Evening Post*, Vol.266, No.2 (March–April) pp.34 (2).

10 Spirduso, W.W. and Eckert, H.M. (1989) The Academy Papers: Physical Activity and Ageing. *Human Kinetics*, Illinois.

Chapter 3

*B*ecoming an effective exercise instructor

f you are genuinely concerned about enhancing older peoples' quality of life, and you are willing to learn the basic exercise principles, if you are sensitive, positive, open-minded and you have a good sense of humour – then you already have the most important qualities for becoming an effective instructor.

Knowledge and skills

A sound knowledge of basic exercise principles means an instructor can safely and confidently tailor exercises to suit the individual, add appropriate moves and eliminate unsafe practices. Whilst this book aims to provide a foundation for guidance required to meet the physical activity needs of older people, it can not cover everything you need to know. A suitable training course will provide a thorough understanding of basic exercise principles and guidelines for safe and effective classes. But even when you are qualified you will still have much to learn and you will need to be constantly up to date.

You can contact the Local Health Education office, Sports Council or YMCA for infor-

mation on relevant workshops, seminars, and training courses (also see Chapter 4 and the Resources section in this book). For a wider view of issues affecting older people, take a look at subjects such as nutrition, psychology, gerontology, anthropology and physiology. This information is available in your local library, GP surgery or university libraries. Exchange information and forge links with other health professionals such as nurses, doctors, physiotherapists and alternative practitioners who can provide further support, ideas and advice.

Communication

Sharing knowledge and information with colleagues is a vital step to creating a network of support which in turn helps and encourages others to increase their rehabilitative role. Talking about exercise can foster a positive attitude which can be communicated to older people in care. Often, there is the temptation to talk to older people as if they were children. Older people are mature, intelligent adults with unique personalities and backgrounds. Find out about each resident's background, interests, past roles and family. This information can then be matched to the activities programme. For example, Dorothy tells me she 'can't stand' the Max Bygrave 'sing-a-long' tunes I often play in my classes, Dorothy prefers classical music, particularly Mozart. So we agreed we would keep a few Max Bygrave songs in the programme since others do enjoy them, but the relaxation period would include music from Dorothy's Mozart collection.

Observation

Of course, exercise leaders need to constantly observe class members to make sure moves are performed properly to avoid injury. But careful observation can provide other kinds of information and increase awareness of an individuals needs, moods and comfort level. Body language and facial expressions in particular can be very useful. Someone in trouble might display an obvious pained expression, or the signs may be more subtle, clenched jaw, tense brow etc. But some people show no altered facial signs or body language, a class member may instead give up or refuse to join in because they are in pain, frustrated or depressed. Careful observation can help to uncover such problems so that appropriate adjustments can be made to the class, making it safe and meaningful for each person.

Expectations

If there is the feeling that nursing and residential homes are just places where you go to die, then what is the point in taking exercise? Narrow expectations of older people is one of the biggest obstacles to conquer – and some stereotypes persist. Society seems to expect older people to be sedentary. Many people still think older people have completed their 'useful' lives. The really terrible thing is that many older people hold these same expectations of themselves. This is not surprising when this generation is regularly told: 'put your feet up', 'you shouldn't be doing that at your age'. Gradually activity is decreased, energy and strength is lost and the person is no longer able to move independently.

Humour

We have all heard that laughter is the best medicine. The Bible tells us of the positive benefit of humour – 'A cheerful heart does good like a medicine: but a broken spirit makes one sick' (Proverbs 17:22). Certainly a jolly good laugh has many benefits (Table 3.1). The really good news is that it is costs nothing and is almost certainly the only medicine without harmful side effects. Just as food nourishes our bodies, laughter nourishes our spirit and is as basic a need as shelter, warmth and love. It also has the power to communicate acceptance and deepen the holistic caring role.

Although humour can promote well being, sometimes the health care worker may in fact create communication obstacles by trying to 'jolly up' someone. This can happen if older individuals feel that their problems have been minimized or not taken seriously. Personal criticism, insults, sarcasm and humour which uses racial prejudice or reinforces negative stereotypical images have no place in any caring relationship and if used may only increase stress, anxiety and isolation. Yet, there is also a danger that spontaneous interaction may be lost and humour deliberately avoided by the overcautious carer nervous about hurting someone's feelings.

Table 3.1 The benefits of humour

A good laugh:

- Is 'infectious'
- Releases endorphins (the body's own natural painkillers)
- Relieves stress and anxiety
- Increases the heart rate, circulation and oxygen intake
- Exercises chest and lungs
- Helps to create a new frame of reference – 'puts things into perspective'

Following a good laugh:

- Muscles become more relaxed and tension is eased
- Heart and breathing rates decrease
- Mood, confidence and self-esteem are raised
- Positive social interaction is encouraged
- Important messages are communicated

The beneficial effects of humour include the relief of stress and anxiety. A jolly good laugh increases the heart rate, circulation and oxygen intake. Heart and breathing rates decrease following laughter, muscles become more relaxed and tension is eased. Pain may also be reduced as a result of distraction, lowered tension and the release of endorphins – the body's natural painkillers. Promoting activity for older people is a serious concern,

but the older people I work with tell me they come to my class because they can also 'forget their troubles' and 'have some fun'.

Table 3.2 How to include humour into our daily lives

- Share something good that happened to you recently and ask others for their experiences (this can be something like a visit from a loved one, a letter from a friend or simply waking up to the sound of birds singing)
- Imagine you are happy for no reason at all
- Find a cartoon in a newspaper or magazine and make up an alternative caption
- Write to or telephone a friend you have been meaning to contact
- Exercise, stretch or deep breathe to release 'happy hormones' in the brain (natural endorphins)
- Do not feel guilty about being happy and do not think you will have to 'pay for it later' – we do not always have to earn the right to be happy

Motiviating your students

I have to admit that motivating some people to exercise can be quite a challenge, and not all older people will be keen to increase their activities or join in an exercise session. Many people are happy to have everything done for them, or they may underestimate their physical abilities, seeing exercise as an activity for younger people only. They may feel a little shy or think 'it's too late to start now'. Sometimes those with physical limitations feel uncomfortable in the company of others, especially if they think they will be unable to keep up with the rest of the class. Sensitive enquiries may however help to understand more about each individual's earlier lifestyles, and reveal similarities between individuals that can be included when structuring group activity programmes. The challenge is not to insist that everyone joins in an activity class, but rather to encourage participation by helping people to understand the benefits.

Know your student

Although the idea of exercise is often well accepted by older people, many of those new to the idea of structured exercise tend to see it as something for others and not for themselves. They may say things like 'I'm too old for that kind of thing now' or 'my legs are no good anymore'. These attitudes take time to change, but working closely with older people allows us to understand each resident's personality, habits and health position so we

can find the correct approach. For example, if I know a resident is not sleeping well, we talk about how exercise and relaxation can help to prepare the mind and body for a good night's sleep. Activity is more likely to be increased when the person sees exercise as rewarding.

Goal setting and encouragement

Motivation is increased with support, reassurance and encouragement. An effective exercise leader recognises all progress, no matter how small. Try to reward individual exercise efforts and respect participants' enthusiasm, intelligence, abilities, limitations, and experience. Encourage short term goals which can be fairly quickly achieved, such as posture improvement. Also be specific when agreeing on the amount of

Figure 3.1 Using a wall calendar (adapted from Get Ready to Exercise[2])

OCTOBER		
Mrs Emma Martin Goal – to exercise for 10–15 minutes a day		
1 Shoulder Shrugs × 4 Circling Arms × 4 Shoulder Stretch Rocking Feet × 4 Foot Circles × 4 Chair Push up × 1 Deep Breathing and Relaxation (12)	2 Shoulder Shrugs × 4 Circling Arms × 4 Upward Stretch × 4 Tropicana Wiggle × 4 Foot Circles × 4 Chair Push up × 2 Deep Breathing and Relaxation (15)	3 Circling Arms × 4 Back Stroke × 4 Piano Playing Head Press × 4 Vocal Vowels × 4 Tropicana Wiggle × 4 Foot Circles × 4 Sit to Stand × 1 Deep Breathing (14)
8	9	10

Record total time spent exercising in brackets

exercise to commit to on a daily basis. It is no use just agreeing to exercise regularly – this is too general and easy to ignore or forget. Each individual will have an idea of the amount of exercise they are able to commit to. For example, a plan to exercise for five minutes each morning is an achievable goal to start with. This can be increased with everyone's agreement so that the exercises remain challenging. Use a large wall calendar (Figure 3.1) to record activities, reinforce the idea of daily exercise and help set realistic goals. What is important though is not how quickly a target is reached, but whether or not progress is being made.

Community contact

Many older people I meet have experienced lifelong connections with the community. These connections help to give structure and a sense of purpose to their lives. Major life events such as illness, disability, loss of job, home, friends and family can reduce or completely sever these important connections. Life satisfaction is reduced and people in these situations tell me they feel 'useless to anyone', or 'just a burden'. We all appreciate feeling needed and useful – this is no different for older people. A local residential care home in my area regularly invites nursery school children into the home so they can join in with activity sessions. The older people feel useful and needed as they help the children with play activities, and the children benefit from the older person's experience and personal attention. Getting together for an activity session encourages community spirit within the care home. Individuals may also discover similar interests which promote friendship.

Public relations

A further way of reaching out into the community for support is to invite the local newspaper to write a feature article about the positive efforts older people are making. This becomes a very exciting event which increases the self-esteem and confidence of those participating and may even help to change some of society's negative attitudes about older people. Care home staff and even those who do not participate also enjoy seeing their residential home featured in such a positive way. This is easy to organise. Just call up your local newspaper, who are always looking for good local stories, and invite them to attend an exercise session. I have organised a couple of these events now, and on each occasion the residents and staff had so much fun simply preparing for the event. The photographs appeared in the local newspaper and drew a great deal of attention from the local community, health care staff and residents' families. This positive feeling lasted for weeks and remained a popular topic of conversation long after the event.

Finally, think of what motivates you to exercise or take up a new activity. My own exercise reward is that it helps keep me fit and healthy. Even so, I am often tempted to drop an exercise session because of time constraints or because it simply feels like too much trouble. If the activity is stimulating and challenging I am much more keen to exercise. Manufacturers of exercise equipment are regularly trying to persuade us that exercise can be a positive, fun and rewarding experience. Just look at the vast range of exercise aids and gimmicks out there aimed at capturing our interest. Everyone needs a little help and encouragement to become or remain motivated. Older people are no exception to this.

The special rewards of working with older people

Figures show that we are living longer and the older population (that is those aged 65 or over) has grown twice as fast as the rest of the population during the last two decades. At the turn of the century here in the UK life expectancy was only 48 years for men and 52 years for women. By the 1990s, lifespan had increased by a dramatic 50 per cent bringing a life expectancy of 72 for men and 77 for women. Within this group of people it is the oldest who are living longer. By the year 2025, it is estimated that there will be two million people over the age of 80 in the UK[1].

We cannot stop the clock, but we can help stop expectations that promote a sedentary lifestyle for older people. A growing interest in exercise and positive living for older people is helping to debunk old myths that reinforce negative attitudes and beliefs, such as: 'older people should take it easy' and 'exercise is for young people'. Those of us who work closely with older people have a unique opportunity to help improve the lives of this rapidly growing segment of the population by increasing their physical activity levels.

The challenge of ageism

Very often, society and older people themselves unquestionably accept loss of function, illness and disability as a natural consequence of ageing. We place high value on youth and beauty but growing old holds many negative images. Think of all the 'anti-ageing' creams and potions out there that claim to interrupt the 'ravages of old age', make you look ten years younger and reduce 'ugly wrinkles' and 'age spots'. It is these images that help to perpetuate ageism which in turn treats older people as one amorphous group.

As exercise leaders working with older people, we must question our own attitudes about ageing and ask how they affect the people we work with. How do we see ourselves as older people? Do we see only years of illness and disability ahead or do we see ourselves as active, mature individuals in control of a future filled with opportunity?

Particular rewards

The rewards of working with older people are so much greater when our efforts address the deeper issues of daily living activity and independence. Even those frail older people who have been inactive for many years can benefit from a supervised programme of exercises that explores, develops and maximises the potential to lead healthier, more active and involved lives. At the very least, we are talking about exercises that older people themselves describe as making them 'feel better'. The alternative choice is one of inactivity which must undoubtedly condemn older people in our care to a life of increasing decrepitude.

I would like to tell you about a few of my personal reward experiences from working with older people who are in care.

Harry and Mae

Harry and Mae had been married for over 60 years and had decided to move into a care home when successive attacks of bronchitis and arthritic flare ups had left them both quite frail and weak. They encouraged each other to come to the exercise classes and always attended together. Harry had a wonderful voice and enjoyed singing along to the music we played in class. Mae's health quickly deteriorated and she died after quite a short illness. Harry was devastated and stayed away from class for several months. I would visit Harry and just let him know that the exercise group was thinking of him and that we missed his lovely voice. Gradually Harry renewed his interest in the classes and began once again to join in. He would get very tearful but still managed to sing along with the tunes. Other class members were very caring and it was clear that Harry found this support comforting. Whilst Harry remained very sad about his loss, he began to look forward to and enjoy the classes.

Muriel

Muriel was a resident in a nursing home because chronic and severe arthritis had left her with many disabilities and she was no longer able to care for herself at home. Muriel was well versed with her condition and treatment but was always searching for additional ways to help herself. The social co-ordinator at the care home approached me to ask if Muriel would be a good candidate for the activity sessions. I visited Muriel and we talked about exercise and arthritis. She told me that she had always been advised to rest, and I agreed that this was certainly the best thing to do with inflamed and painful joints, but that when these painful episodes had passed – exercise could help to nourish and strengthen the joints. Gradually we started an exercise plan consisting of just five minutes of simple finger

and toe exercises to be carried out twice a day. She found that these exercises were easier to do when she was in the bath, the warm water supporting and soothing her hands. Once she gained confidence and felt comfortable with these moves she agreed to join in the class. Muriel told me the exercises decreased the stiffness in her joints and even more importantly to her, she was able to feel more in control of her arthritis.

Glenda

Glenda also suffered from arthritis and joint stiffness, and as her carers said, she was 'very fragile'. Glenda told me she was 'too weak' to exercise. I knew Glenda used to play the church organ so I had an idea she would enjoy listening to the music we played in our exercise sessions. She was pleased to have been invited to listen to the music but told me that she really could not join in. Yet she did participate – in her own way. The music obviously helped to inspire Glenda to move and she would mime piano playing movements with her fingers. Over the weeks her 'piano playing' became more vigorous and she would use her whole body to move. Glenda told me her 'tail end' did not seem as sore since joining the classes. This was music to my ears!

■ Exercises should be started slowly and maintained at a comfortable pace

■ A few minutes of simple moves once – or if possible – twice a day

■ Repeat the sets to increase time spent exercising

■ An exercise habit is encouraged if exercises are carried out at approximately the same time each day

- Exercises can also be enjoyed whilst in the bath

- In times of illness or discomfort exercise should be postponed

References

1 Laing, W. and Hall, M. (1991) *Demographic Trends – Agenda for Health: The Challenges of Ageing.* Association of the British Pharmaceutical Industry, London.

2 Fiatarone, M.A. (1994) *Get Ready To Exercise! (Part 2: Endurance Training).* Fit For Your Life Research Studies Center, Boston, MA.

Chapter 4

Safety first

Susie Dinan

How can we get more older people more active for more of the time, safely and effectively? How can we balance increased activity amongst older people with safety and effectiveness? This is the dilemma facing all health and exercise professionals involved in the promotion, management and delivery of physical activity programmes for older people.

In 1990, the safety aspects of this challenge were highlighted when Dr Roy Shephard pointed out that programming physical activity for older participants requires more care and more expertise than for any other group, with only a fine line separating effective from dangerous procedures[1]. Pausing to consider any group of older exercisers confirms the validity of this observation. Such a group is likely to have a high proportion of participants with some form of disability or one or more chronic illnesses. Physical activity, fitness levels and functional capacity are also likely to be lower than in younger individuals. All of these aspects are likely to be more marked in chair class participants. Personal goals are also diverse; some participants want a vigorous, continuous workout whilst others happily drop out after the warm up, only joining in again for the après class tea and chat, if not encouraged through every move. For some participants just sitting with the group each week may be enough initially.

It is this unique interrelationship between the ageing process, wide ranging fitness and activity levels, disease, disability, belief systems and personal goals that narrows the safety margins when programming exercise for the older person. It is essential therefore to ensure that risks are reduced to a minimum.

Prevention is a priority

Although there is no way to eliminate the risks completely, education and guidance of the participants and professionals involved can eliminate most of the hazards[2]. Later chapters concentrate on the design (content and structure) and the delivery (coaching) of the exercise session. This chapter provides practical safety guidelines for the Chair Leader or Exercise Instructor, as well as for the participant. It will enable all concerned to work towards achieving sound, evidence based approaches that meet individual participants' health needs, functional interests and means. The chapter also considers ways of creating safer environments and provides an exercise and fitness education and training perspective. In addition, it gives guidelines for building professional relationships and adapting exercise for some of the most common chronic diseases and disabilities found in older people.

It is tempting to think that these cautionary messages need not apply to chair exercise. But even though it is true that many hazards are greatly reduced (and in some instances eliminated) in a well designed and delivered chair session, certain exercises must still be excluded and others adapted for specific problems.

The safety precautions and guidelines that follow apply equally to chair and standing exercise. For example, both participant and instructor need to be clear about the particular aims, adaptations and cautions for each individual. They should also be conversant with the body 'signs' indicating when exercise should be stopped, when it can continue and when it is best avoided. Getting to know participants, having a good rapport with them before, during and after sessions, as well as keeping up to date with current exercise thinking, are key factors in keeping risks to a minimum.

Preparation

Before the start of sessions, chair leaders/ exercise instructors should take time to:

- identify participants with chronic diseases and disabilities, and seek medical advice where appropriate

- assess current physical activity levels and previous exercise history

- identify activities that are appropriate for the whole group

- ensure that they can adapt the exercise appropriately for each individual, for example providing support for 'sit to stand' for someone with knee pain

- ensure that they can recognise and respond to signs of distress and are familiar with emergency procedures

- ensure that participants are taught how to recognise and respond appropriately to the effects of exercise

- ensure that the environment is conducive to safe, comfortable exercise

- establish working relationships with a range of health professionals

So, before beginning, there are some important checks and preparations to be made.

Step 1 – First a health check

In order for exercise programmes to be safe and individually tailored, a written health assessment should be carried out for all individuals, whatever their age and health status. This should cover all relevant health factors and should be completed before the exercise programme is begun.

Although there are very real concerns about the over medicalisation of recreational activities, as it may imply that exercise is a risky business, much of this can be put to positive use. It is important to make clear (both to health professionals and to participants themselves) that the idea is not to ensure safety by exclusion, but rather to ensure inclusion at an appropriate level.

Checking with your doctor before starting exercise after many years of inactivity can be positively promoted when it is presented as a simple, commonsense measure. It is in fact recommended by the American College of Sports Medicine (ACSM) for all individuals over the age of 35[3].

Frailer, older individuals require even more thorough preparation. At present there is a lamentable lack of uniformity in the guidelines relating to pre-exercise assessment procedures for all older participants. However several respected authorities have recommended a customised health and ageing assessment questionnaire for everyone over 69 years of age[3,4]. Instructors of older participants should ensure that their new recruits seek advice from their doctor about any relevant health problems or risk factors prior to starting exercise. In particular, they should seek medical advice if they have:

- been told at any time that they have heart trouble, or if they are being treated for any heart condition

- had a heart attack in the last three years

- chest pain while at rest and/or during exertion

- faintness, dizziness and/or fast, irregular or very slow heart beats

- high blood pressure

- had diabetes for more than ten years

- shortness of breath after exertion and sometimes even at rest or at night in bed

- had a fracture of the hip, spine or wrist, at any time during adulthood

- had a fall more than twice (no matter what the reason) during the last year

- arthritis or a joint problem

- pain in the buttocks, backs of legs, thighs or calves on walking

- swollen ankles, feet, hands and/or take diuretics (water tablets)

- any lacerated wounds or cuts on the feet that are slow to heal

- done no regular activity for three years or more and are over 69

- the intention of taking up vigorous exercise.

As one or more of the above will apply to many older people, it is not surprising that a growing number of experts recommend that all older participants have a check-up (to include standing and lying blood pressure readings) before beginning any exercise programme. This health check can also act as a 'baseline' against which all the parties involved (the instructor, the doctor and the participant) can measure improvement. The Pre-exercise Questionnaire in the Appendix at the end of this chapter is a useful model for the exercise professional. It should be looked at in conjunction with the Guidelines that follow it.

Step 2 – Optional safety check

Self assessment

Including some self-assessment indicators (see below) as part of the health assessment provides an important insight into the person's performance of everyday actions. It also gives an opportunity to learn more about their current and past activity levels and interests, personal approaches, and anything that may act as a barrier to physical activity. For example, if you want to gauge the functional capabilities of your participants, the following '50+ All to Play For' questions are a useful starting point[4].

How unfit are you?

- Are you left gasping for breath even if you run or walk only a short distance (e.g. 50 yards)?

- Does your heart thump after climbing a few flights of stairs?

- Do you ache all over after digging a small patch of garden?

- Are you tired out after doing an hour of housework?

- Are you tired out after carrying two bags of shopping for a short distance?

- Is it an effort to bend and tie your shoe laces?

- What is the most energetic activity you are used to?

'Yes' in answer to any of these questions

means the participant probably leads a sedentary life and is unused to any exercise. Such participants will need to start with mobility and flexibility exercises and very gentle strength and stamina work. Vigorous activity should not be attempted.

Assessment through observation

Careful observation during warm up exercises and normal movements (such as sit to stand, walking across the room, etc.) provides valuable insights into both physical capabilities and accuracy of the self assessment. These familiar, task-oriented approaches also have the advantage of 'demedicalising' the whole process and relating it firmly to life. Dawn Skelton's *Functional Assessment*[5] provides useful further reading.

Functional assessments also provide an opportunity to introduce the participant to basic exercise techniques and information about the benefits of exercise in old age; both can assist in greater safety and motivation. Importantly, these preparation steps provide an invaluable opportunity to get to know the person on several levels.

Adopting a conversational tone can help to keep the assessment process 'person focused' rather than paper focused. The questions are merely a checklist to ensure consistency of information and approach by the exercise professional. The aim is to gain as clear a picture of the exercise needs as possible prior to participation.

Step 3 – Day-to-day preparation

Just as important as getting to know participants in the pre-exercise assessment is making time to welcome them (each and every one) before each session. Simply making eye contact can be an instructive way of gauging how someone feels that day. Sensitivity in exploring this before the session starts, together with watching participants closely during the warm up, may point to a complete change in the way the session for that day needs to be delivered. Requesting additional assistance, explicitly advising an individual to take it easy, or even stopping the session temporarily, are some of the many strategies required to meet the fluctuating health and functional status of frail groups. It is essential to respond to the situation on a day by day, minute by minute basis.

In the rest home, day centre or ward setting this preparation or 'health handover' can be achieved particularly effectively provided it is part of the care setting schedule. Before the class, the instructor should check the patients' notes and consult the staff in charge. Making sure that staff understand the contraindictions to exercise will help them to hand over relevant information, and to make informed decisions with the instructor about individuals' suitability to participate. Many a well-meaning staff member or carer has brought a patient with a temperature, a chest infection or an acutely inflamed leg to an exercise session, thinking it would do no harm. Similarly, if anything happens during the session to cause concern, it is important to do a verbal handover with senior staff and put a written record in the relevant notes or notebook. Passing information on to other exercise colleagues involved (whilst observing the usual confidentiality procedures) is also important.

Exercise: when to stop and when to continue

Part of the preparation process must be to ensure that participants have clear guidelines as to when exercise should be stopped or when it may be continued. For example, a person with arthritis should discontinue any exercise where an increase in pain lasts longer than two hours. It should also be remembered that pain may not occur until the following day (see page 41 for further information). Again participants must be taught the importance of excluding themselves from participation when they are unwell. And teachers must reinforce this message.

Warning signs

Participants should be temporarily excluded from exercise or encouraged to stop and seek advice if:

- they have a high temperature, chest or other respiratory infection

- they have been vomiting, or are experiencing diarrhoea, dizziness, extreme fatigue, unstable diabetes or acute kidney disease

- there is uncharacteristic swelling in their extremities

- they feel unwell.

Participants should also be taught in advance to recognise and respond immediately and confidently to symptoms of distress experienced once exercise is under way. Indications that exercise is too stressful and should be stopped immediately are:

- pain or discomfort in the chest, abdomen, back, neck, jaw or arms

- undue swelling

- extreme pallor, especially around the mouth

- sweating combined with pallor

- cold sweat

- extreme and unfamiliar shortness of breath

- irregular heart beat

- confusion, unfamiliar loss of attention

- dizziness, fainting or tripping while exercising

- a nauseous sensation during or after exercise

- pain in one or both of the legs

- pain in the joints or anywhere in the body

- extreme fatigue

- extreme stiffness lasting more than two days.

Knowing when to continue exercise is also important. The clearer both participant and instructor are about comfort while exercising, the safer, more effective and more enjoyable the exercises will be. Giving tangible, specific indicators of appropriate responses to exercise will also increase participants' confidence and independence in assessing whether they are working too hard or not hard enough. Knowing what to expect while exercising is reassuring; with practice and feedback even over ambitious or over cautious participants can learn to work more effectively and safely.

Continue signs

Indications that exercise is just about right are:

- breathing a little more than usual

- feeling warmer (too hot in normal clothing) even sweating a little

- feeling that the muscles are working more than usual (a mild pulling sensation during the stretches, beginning to feel warm, tired, or even a slight 'burning' sensation during the strength exercises).

Mild stiffness the following day is normal if a person is starting from scratch or starting a new strength exercise, but severe stiffness is a sign of having overdone it.

Additional safety messages

Giving accurate information about the benefits of specific types and or amounts of exercise is an important function for all health and exercise professionals. It can dispel myths that can adversely affect both participation and safety. Most importantly accurate advice empowers older people to make informed activity choices (see Chapter 5 for further information on amounts of exercise). Other helpful pointers and safety messages to get across in this preparation phase and again during participation include the following:

- There is no gain where there is pain or strain; there is a difference between discomfort and pain.

- Quality is more important than quantity.

- Breathing should be regular and natural. Never hold the breath.

- Exercise, like medicine, has moved on in recent years – head circles and toe touching have been replaced by sounder, more effective solutions.

- Strength training is quite safe if performed correctly. It will not only strengthen bone and muscle but will also help to improve balance, walking speed, stair climbing power, body warmth and ability to withstand illness. It will not build unsightly muscles.

- Breathing and heart rate will increase a little; this is how we get fit. If you can pass the talk test by chatting comfortably to a friend for a few seconds then you've got the pace just about right.

- Once a week is better than nothing but it is better to do something every day rather than a long session once a week. A total of 30 minutes moderate activity nearly every day will bring optimal benefits[2] (see Chapter 5 for further details).

- It is never too late to begin.

Step 4 – Safer, more effective, more enjoyable spaces

A functional environment can play a surprisingly effective part in promoting safety. It is an important part of the exercise professional's responsibilities to provide such an environment. Setting up prior to the session takes time and energy but is well worth the effort. A well organised, clean, attractive and clutter free space with interesting, well maintained equipment indicates a level of professional care that is appreciated by participants and staff. Preparation can often set the tone for the group. If the space looks inviting and interesting then resistance to

moving from easy chairs to straight-backed exercise chairs – or just moving at all – is minimised. A well lit, airy space with a large, bright ball in the centre of a circle of chairs, colourful resistance bands placed across each chair, water jug and cups at the ready and a Scottish reel playing in the background are hard to resist[6].

Additional considerations

Other points to consider include the following:

- Chairs should be sturdy and straight backed, with comfortable flat seats (and preferably no arms).

- There should be easy toilet access.

- The floor should be clean and free from obstacles.

- In multipurpose spaces, furniture should be moved and safely stored.

- Tissues, water and cups and litter bin need to be available.

- Equipment must be checked – for example, for holes in resistance bands. Anything needing replacement or repair should be reported.

- The area to be used should be well ventilated, but also warm and draught free.

- The area needs to be well lit, preferably by daylight or a combination of daylight and artificial light – avoid direct sunlight.

- There must be a telephone within easy access.

- Emergency drills need to be in place.

- First aid kits must be well stocked and accessible.

- Participants will need to wear comfortable clothing and supportive, flattish shoes.

- Safe access to and from the session (handrail, personal escort etc.) may need to be arranged.

Special safety considerations for chair work[7]

The choice, condition and transfer of the chair involve some important safety considerations. The benefits of chair work mean that the following detailed pointers are entirely worth the extra effort.

Height

The chair back and the chair seat need to be an appropriate height for each individual to ensure an upright, supported posture and unrestricted circulation. The knees need to be at a right angle to the hips, and positioned directly over the ankle. The feet must be in contact with the floor. In order to achieve this alignment in smaller and taller people, it may be necessary to use additional equipment. A telephone directory placed under the feet of a smaller person or on the chair seat for a taller person is a handy solution. Where chair-supported standing work is possible, select higher backed chairs for taller people[6]. Using the wall for support may be an appropriate option.

Weight

The chair should be sturdy, i.e. neither so light and flimsy that it slides or tips, nor so heavy that it could cause injury.

Shape

It is essential to aim for armless, straight-backed chairs with as comfortable and flat a seat as possible. Large foam blocks or firm cushions (not soft pillows) can be used to support the spine.

Repair

Chairs must not be used if they have splinters or rough edges. They should be hygienic and in good repair.

Clothing

Loose comfortable skirts, trousers or leggings should be worn – no tight skirts or wide legged trousers. Shoes with heels, open toes or slingbacks, slipperettes and bare feet should be discouraged and replaced by flattish, supportive footwear wherever possible[6].

Teaching

If you are working in a circle format, ensure that all chairs are evenly spaced to avoid 'blind spots' for instructor and participants. This affects enjoyment as well as safety and effectiveness. If you are teaching from the middle of the circle, be sure that you change the way you face frequently. If you are working with one particular individual, take care not to block the rest of the group from your view – anything could happen and you may be too late to respond. If you are using 'right' and 'left' instructions, remember that people on the other side of a circle will perceive you to be moving in the opposite direction. Where going in the same direction matters for safety, getting all members of the group to wave their right hands first works well.

When changing from one spatial format to another (for example, from a circle to a line or if you are clearing space to do standing or walking activities) ensure that each chair is removed to a safe place. Bumping into chairs unexpectedly can reduce confidence as well as cause accidents. If participants are sufficiently able to lift objects, ensure that they have the technique to do this safely[6].

Step 5 – Effective professional relationships

Good professional relationships help to reduce risks and lead to safer, more tailored, exercise and care plans.

The GP, practice nurse, community and psychiatric nursing teams, the physiotherapist, occupational therapist, health visitor, hospital and day centre staff, residential care staff and sheltered housing wardens, are the main professionals involved in the community health care of older people. Good relationships are built up slowly, but prove their worth by providing a supportive network for the older person and for the exercise professional[4,7].

Respecting boundaries

It is important that chair leaders and exercise instructors observe professional boundaries closely. For example, they must make it clear to class participants and health care professionals that they are not medically trained and may need assistance to assess some older individuals' suitability to undertake standard or adapted exercises. They may also need help to adapt certain exercises appropriately, and to decide when particular activities should be avoided. This might include resisted twisting actions for participants with arthritis in the fingers, for example. The health professionals will also need to point out any movements that have been found to place an individual at risk, for example it is essential for chair leaders and exercise instructors to be informed if a participant suffers from dizziness on standing. Again, passing on tips for communicating with someone who has cognition problems can make all the difference to that person's enjoyment of exercise.

Chair leaders and other exercise professionals must also be clear about professional boundaries in their day-to-day actions. For example, they should offer advice on exercise matters only. If a participant feels pain, the exercise professional should refer the person immediately for a medical opinion. Where the exercise teacher is also a nurse, physiotherapist or doctor then the exercise programme can be monitored and adjusted accordingly, so long as the usual ethical and referral protocols are observed.

Maintaining trust

Always ensure that any advice given by health professionals is followed. If you do not agree with or understand the advice, it is important to discuss this fully with the person concerned until you are agreed on the way forward (see pages 131–135). Liaison of this sort can also be an opportunity to inform health professionals what exercise can and cannot achieve; what the exercise teacher can and cannot do, knows and does not know. Honesty is always the best policy. In addition to ensuring advice is heeded, the exercise professional should never do anything to undermine the respect of the patient for their doctor.

Working in this collaborative way soon identifies several pro-exercise doctors, practice nurses, physiotherapists and centre managers, who can often prove to be one of the most useful resources a chair leader or exercise instructor can have.

Record keeping and monitoring

Well kept records can be surprisingly effective in identifying patients who may be at risk as well as providing useful statistics for evaluation and funding. Attendance, progress, minor illnesses and injuries should be recorded after each session. Any correspondence and advice given in respect of more serious health problems should also be kept on file. Physical changes are particularly apparent in the exercise situation, and any changes in health status – falls, depression, and so on – should be discussed with the individual and followed up appropriately. Record keeping also highlights functional improvement and programme changes. Above all it keeps each person 'fresh' in the mind of the exercise professional and ensures more meaningful tailoring of the exercise.

Confidentiality is essential. In health care settings this is part of everyday practice. However, in fitness and community settings this needs to be highlighted. For example, a suitable secure storage place for records must be located and maintained. It is useful to have a register that includes name, address, telephone number, next of kin, GP, and a short or coded health summary of those participants needing extra attention.

In the ward or rest home setting, notes should be made in the patients' records and (where appropriate) in the medical notes. In addition, the pre and post session hand over with senior staff members and other exercise colleagues is an important method of communicating information. Documenting exercise progress also ensures a presence in the care plan.

Secondary care and community settings

Whatever the setting – fitness or recreation club, fitness centre, community centre, day centre or residential home – it is important to make sure that the management knows exactly what is required and when it is required. Ideally extra hands should be scheduled to assist with getting people safely 'into position' for the session and with the session itself, for example in dementia care settings. In addition, it is productive to ascertain what the centre staff would find helpful to make things run more smoothly. For example, a telephone call 45 minutes beforehand, especially if it is an early morning session, reminds staff of your arrival time and which patients are needed. In centres with busy schedules this appears to be particularly appreciated and is safer and more effective as patients or residents can then be then ready, dressed, breakfasted and alert.

Providing staff training helps to ensure staff are well versed in the aims and outcomes of sessions, as well as how to assist patients during the session. If the session is seen merely as entertainment or as a chance for a staff break, all concerned remain unaware of what effective teamwork can achieve. Scheduling the session a minimum of one hour before or after eating (ensuring the tea trolley is kept well out of sight until the session is finished) and keeping strictly to time wherever possible are all examples of make-or-break practical essentials that teamwork can achieve. A staff training update every six months is also a useful way of keeping enthusiasm and skills tuned up. Training also has personal and educational benefits – even inspiring staff to get active themselves, often for the first time. The value of active health care staff as role models in promoting exercise is discussed in Chapter 5. Including some teaching skills in the staff training provides a useful insight into the fact that, although exercise looks as if it is just lots of fun and very easy to lead, there is in fact a science to designing the sessions and an art to teaching them.

Primary care

In primary care settings, a presentation about the benefits of exercise for older patients appears to be effective. In the Exercise Option of the Primary Care for Older Patients in Camden and Islington Project, piloted in the Hampstead Group Practice and co-ordinated by the Primary Care and Population Sciences Department at the Royal Free and University College Medical School, London, we have found that the more pertinent the presentation, the better. The ideal is for an exercise professional and a primary care professional to co-present case studies on specific patients to their colleagues. Supporting information with research and literature resources is especially valued.

Don't be discouraged if such presentations have to be fitted in months in advance – general practice schedules are tightly packed. Use the time advantageously to liaise with individual practitioners about their patients. This should ensure that you are already part of the bigger practice picture prior to the presentation.

Each of these strategies contributes in a different way to a better exchange of information, which in turn enhances the safety, comfort and enjoyment of exercise for the older participant.

Step 6 – Education and training for exercise professionals

Physical activity with older participants requires specialist coaching skills. Training in the design, delivery, progression and adaptation of exercise is essential to the safety of the older participants. Professor Archie Young has likened the elderly person to an athlete both often performing near their limit[5]. Both groups require extra special coaching skills to ensure they achieve optimal performance.

It is increasingly accepted that the supervision (coaching, teaching, instructing) of physical activity for participants of all ages is a skilled process requiring knowledge based competencies in a range of physical and psychological constructs. It is now recognised that providing physical activity for frailer, older people requires an even higher level of competence and specialist training.

Curriculum development in the area of physical activity and ageing is still in its infancy despite dramatic increases in the older adult population. Consequently many exercise leaders co-ordinating programmes for older people have had to rely primarily on self study and 'on the job' training. However there have been rapid developments in recent years. In the UK a vocational training approach has been emphasised, with the provision of recognised, graded, accessible training routes and quality assurance standards. In contrast, the focus in the USA has been on developing graduate level programmes.

In the UK, National Occupational Standards (NOS) now exist which describe the knowledge base and practical competencies that exercise and fitness instructors must possess for teaching general populations. These are sited at Level 2 (the Basic Instruction Certificate). The teaching of exercise and fitness to specialist populations requiring adapted exercise – such as older people or disabled people – is sited at Level 3 NOS (the Advanced Instruction Certificate).

This specialised and advanced level requires understanding of how ageing and medical conditions affect exercise performance and participation. Most importantly, it requires competence in applying this understanding in practice. An integral part of all training routes is the consideration of socio-economic, psychological and lifestyle factors as they impact on physical activity and ageing. Communication skills and Health and Safety issues are also studied. Current CPR and First Aid qualifications are essential requirements at all instructor levels. At the advanced level, all these curriculum aspects are covered in more detail. Where even higher levels of care and competence are required (eg cardiac rehabilitation or falls prevention[7,8,9]) further training has now been established and will eventually come within the NOS Level 3 framework.

Chair exercise

Where then do health care assistants working with frailer older people, but without a formal exercise qualification, fit in? These professionals have the most continued access to this vulnerable group, yet they are often only interested, at least initially, in chair work and perhaps daily walking. In many cases they have been taking chair sessions for many years. Significantly, health care assistants have been the most proactive of all health care professionals in requesting recognised training in gentle exercise.

In order to respond to this unmet training need, Merton, Sutton & Wandsworth and Canterbury & Thanet Health Authorities, together with Camden Leisure Services, the Royal Free and University College School of Medicine, Leicester College and independent advisers have all collaborated to design, pilot, develop and approve a Chair Exercise Leadership module. The Department of Health studied the development phase of this initiative. The module aims to train competence in leading a set combination of 18 chair based exercises. It has been running for two years with great success and is now widely available. Successful candidates wishing to undertake further training to teach more dynamic and/or vigorous activity, such as supported or unsupported standing/travelling exercises for older people, exercise to music, use of weights, circuits etc. will need to undertake the Basic Instructor Certificate and then the Advanced Exercise for the Older Person Instructor Certificate. This route is described in the *EXA Directory*[10], which also lists recognised training providers, and the Department of Health National Quality Assurance Framework for Exercise Referral Systems[11].

Far from restricting practice or 'cloning' exercise approaches, the establishment of national standards seeks to empower both the group leader (with considerable experience but no formal training in exercise or ageing), and the NOS Level 2 exercise instructor, to further their professional development by undertaking recognised, specialist training in exercise for the older person. This drive for excellence is motivated by a need to ensure the greatest possible safety and comfort for vulnerable participants.

Finally and importantly, at every level in England the exercise professional should be registered with The Fitness Alliance (see Resource section)[11]. Registered instructors are properly qualified and insured, and work to a code of ethics and professional practice. Similar registration schemes are run by Fitness Scotland and Fitness Wales.

Future perspectives

So graded, nationally recognised professional development in the area of physical activity and ageing in the UK is established and expanding. For those who wish to take it further, there are graduate level programmes at Stirling and Bristol Universities which have pioneered the integration of physical activity in ageing in physical education. Much still needs to be done however to establish physical activity as important subject matter in the fields of gerontology and primary care. At the other end of the training continuum there is a need for greater access to physical activity promotion programmes for other professional groups already working with older people. For example Senior Peer Mentor Programmes are currently being developed in collaboration with Age Concern's Active Age Unit. These could make a valuable contribution to taking up the challenge of getting more older people more active more often.

Conclusion

The ultimate goal must be to improve health and quality of life through increasing levels of physical activity safely and effectively thereby assisting the older person to maintain health gains for as long as possible. This requires specialist training and knowledge of the ageing process as it relates to the older body's response to exercise and to training; it also requires the ability to apply this knowledge to the planning, delivery, coaching, progression and monitoring of exercise. Confidence in contacting other health care professionals when adapting exercise for older people with chronic conditions and disabilities beyond the scope of the exercise professional is also relevant to safety issues. Close liaison with health professionals and the older exerciser is central to an integrated health related exercise programme.

A safe, focused environment and a well designed, well taught, varied chair exercise programme (that emphasises moderate amounts and intensities of exercise and accommodates individual needs) can make a significant contribution to health gain. Importantly, it also broadens safety margins for the older exerciser. By starting slowly, building gradually and accumulating exercise in flexible combinations that are part of every day life, it is possible to make lasting and positive changes in activity habits that will impact on health and function at every stage of later life.

Both the older person and the health professional will find that the ability to identify accurate, specific benefits as well as appropriate settings, sessions and exercise professionals, will help them to make more informed choices and recommendations about which activities to pursue.

Continuing education of participants by health and exercise professionals, about the benefits of exercise in the later years, will also enhance enjoyment and foster independence – the ultimate motivators for the older participant.

References

1 Shephard, R.J. (1997) *Ageing, Physical Activity and Health*. Human Kinetics, Champagne, Illinois.

2 Young, A. and Dinan, S. (2000) Active in later life. In McLatchie G, Harries M, Williams C, King J, eds. *ABC of Sports Medicine* 2nd edition. BMJ Books, London.

3 American College of Sports Medicine (1998) Position stand on exercise and physical activity for older adults. *Medicine Science, Sports and Exercise* 30(6): 992–1008.

4 Bassey, J. and Fentem, P. (1990) *50+ All to Play For*. Sports Council, London.

5 Skelton, D. (1998) Validated Functional Assessment Tests. In Simey P, Pennington B, eds. *Physical Activity and the Prevention and Management of Falls and Accidents among older people. A Framework for Practice*. Health Education Authority, London.

6 Dinan, S. (1998) Fit for Life: Why exercise is vital for everyone. *Journal of Dementia Care*, 6(3):22–25.

7 Dinan, S. and Skelton, D. (2000) *Exercise for the Prevention of Falls and Injuries. A Specialist Training Course Manual for Health and Exercise Professionals*. Leicester College. Leicester.

8 Bell, J. *et al.* (1997) *British Association of Cardiac Rehabilitation: Exercise Instructor Training Module*. British Heart Foundation, London.

9 Dinan, S. (2000) *Chair Exercise Leadership Training Course Manual for Health and Exercise Professionals Working with Frailer, Older People*. Leicester College, Leicester.

10 Health Education Authority (1998) *The EXA Directory. Courses and qualifications for teaching and instructing in physical activity and exercise*. Health Education Authority, London.

11 Department of Health (2001) *National Quality Assurance Framework for Exercise Referral Systems*. HMSO, London.

Further reading

1 Sharp, C. and Dinan, S.M. (1998) *Fitness for Later Life*. Piatkus Books, London.

2 American College of Sports Medicine (1997) *ACSM's Exercise Management for Persons with Chronic Diseases and Disabilities*. Human Kinetics, Illinois.

3 Dinan, S. and Skelton, D. (2000) *Exercise for the Prevention of Falls and Injuries. A Specialist Training Course Manual for Health and Exercise Professionals*. Leicester College. Leicester.

Appendix – Exercise resources

Pre-exercise questionnaire

This questionnaire has been adapted from work carried out at the Human Nutrition Centre on Aging at Tufts University, Boston. It is recommended that all individuals over the age of 69 complete this, with the help of their doctor *prior to participation in an exercise session*.

Encourage participants to answer each question honestly 'yes' or 'no'. A 'yes' answer to any of the questions requires further discussion with the person's doctor *before* exercising starts.

Pre-exercise questionnaire

	Yes	No
1 Do you get chest pains while at rest and/or during exertion?	☐	☐
2 If the answer to Question 1 is 'yes', is it true that you haven't had a doctor diagnose these pains yet?	☐	☐
3 Have you ever had a heart attack?	☐	☐
4 If the answer to Question 3 is 'yes', was your heart attack within the last year?	☐	☐
5 Do you have high blood pressure?	☐	☐
6 If you don't know the answer to Question 5, answer this: Was your last blood pressure reading more than 150/100?	☐	☐
7 Do you have diabetes?	☐	☐
8 (If the answer to Question 7 is 'yes') Is your diabetes going without treatment at present?	☐	☐
9 Are you short of breath after extremely mild exertion and sometimes even at rest or at night in bed?	☐	☐

		Yes	No
10	Do you have any ulcerated wounds or cuts on your feet that don't seem to heal?	☐	☐
11	Have you unexpectedly lost 10lbs or more in the past six months?	☐	☐
12	Do you get pain in your buttocks, the back of your legs, or in your thighs or calves when you walk?	☐	☐
13	While at rest, do you frequently experience fast irregular heartbeats? Or, at the other extreme, very slow beats? (While a low heart rate can be a sign of an efficient and well-conditioned heart, a very low rate can also indicate a cause for concern.)	☐	☐
14	Are you currently being treated for any heart or circulatory condition, such as vascular disease, stroke, angina, hypertension, congestive heart failure, poor circulation to the legs, valvular heart disease, blood clots, or chest or lung disease?	☐	☐
15	As an adult, have you ever had a fracture of the hip, spine or wrist?	☐	☐
16	Have you had more than two falls in the past year (no matter what the reason)?	☐	☐
17	Are you on any medication? If the answer is 'yes' please list:	☐	☐

....

....

Even if you answered 'No' to all 17 questions, all people over the age of 69 who are about to begin a physical training programme are advised to have a health check.

Your name _____

Address _____ Tel No _____

Contact in Emergency

Name _____

Address _____ Tel No _____

GP _____

Address _____ Tel No _____

	Yes	No
Do you have poor hearing?	☐	☐
Or wear a hearing aid?	☐	☐
Do you have poor eyesight?	☐	☐
Do you have poor eyesight even with glasses?	☐	☐

I have read, understood and completed this questionnaire. Any queries I had were answered to my full satisfaction.

_____   _____   _____

Signature   Date   Witness

I acknowledge my patient's intention to undertake a structured exercise session supervised by qualified, specialised exercise for the older person instructors or chair leaders.

_____   _____

Signature of doctor   Date

Guidelines for adapting exercise for chronic conditions and disabilities common in old age

Aim of the guidelines

The aim of these Guidelines is to assist the exercise leader or instructor working with older people to adapt exercise for a safer more enjoyable experience. They provide a greater understanding of how a selection of the most common diseases found among older people may affect an individual's readiness and response to exercise. Each set of Guidelines follows a common pattern incorporating the following headings:

- Definition

- Main characteristics

- Effects on the exercise response

- Possible effects of medication

- Pre-exercise assessment

- Types of exercise

- Special considerations/precautions

- Aims and benefits of exercise.

It is essential to be aware however that no matter what the condition(s) or disability(ies):

- Each disease is different and individuals will each respond in their own way.

- Many older people have multiple disease problems and medications and do not fit neatly into a single disease approach.

- The person themselves will be the most important source of information on how their movement and performance of daily actions are affected. Where there are cognitive problems, family and professional carers can often assist the person to provide a fuller picture.

- No matter what the condition nearly all older people can benefit from exercise provided the pace is gentle to moderate and progress is slow and cautious.

- The aim is to increase independence and improve enjoyment and quality of life.

- Liaison with health professionals is the key to adapting exercise for individual participants.

Arthritis

Definition

There are over a hundred different sub-types of arthritis, which are classified under two main types.

OA (osteoarthritis)

A localised, progressive joint disease that is characterised by degeneration of the cartilage that lines the joint, and/or the formation of osteophytes within the joint capsule. Osteoarthritis is confined to hands, spine, knees and hips. It affects 30 per cent of older people.

RA (rheumatoid arthritis)

An inflammatory multi-joint, multi-system disease. Rheumatoid arthritis is characterised by inflammation of the synovial membrane of the joint(s). It usually takes the form of recurrent attacks that result in progressive deterioration of the joint. It is an autoimmune disease and also affects many other organs of the body. It is found in many joints – wrists, hands, knees, feet, cervical spine. Rheumatoid arthritis affects all ages, but particularly women aged between 30–40.

Main characteristics

- OA – 'Local' joint pain, stiffness, bone spurs (osteophytes), cartilage breakdown. Hot and slightly red, increased stickiness of the joint lubricant (synovial fluid).

- RA – 'Systemic' chronic multi-joint pain, severe stiffness, acute and chronic inflammation, fusing of bone ends, breakdown of cartilage and synovial membrane and loss of joint structure. Hot, red, inflamed, increased stickiness of synovial fluid.

Effects on exercise response

- Acute flare up blunts the person's response to exercise. Only mobility, gentle stretching and rest are recommended during this phase.

- Effects are worse in the morning.

- Range of movement may be severely restricted.

- Pain and stiffness increases energy cost of all activity by as much as 50 per cent.

- Poor ability to perform repetitive, rapid actions such as marching.

- Site and severity determine exercise choices.

- People with joint disease tend to be more de-conditioned and therefore more at risk.

- In RA be aware of additional effects on cardiovascular, respiratory systems, etc.

- Possible effects of medication include:
    - anaemia
    - peripheral neuropathy (altered sensation in the extremities, usually feet)
    - osteoporosis
    - obesity in trunk.

Pre-exercise assessment

- It is essential to establish the type, site(s) and severity of the arthritis.

- Establish current functional capacity in the affected joints. Give functional tasks such as holding equipment, sit to stand, upward reaching, to identify specific limitations.

- Orthotics are often needed to assist participation.

Types of exercise

- Non-weight bearing or minimal weight-bearing.

- Longer warm up and warm down needed.

- Mobility and stretching exercises first.

- Water exercise for preference; hydrotherapy wherever possible.

- Endurance: use support – wall or chair; do only one minute to begin, monitor, then progress very cautiously in the early stages.

- Strengthening exercises for joint support. Ensure that a chair or cushion supports the spine. Always use static muscle contractions (held still) at first; introduce one exercise at a time around the affected area and only one repetition at first. Build up gradually to six repetitions before introducing other exercises around the affected area. Discontinue if there are any adverse effects. Finally progress to isotonic muscle contraction (eg moving the resistance band as far apart as possible then returning it in a controlled way to where it started).

Special considerations/cautions

- RA – peripheral neuropathy.

- RA – eye and other tissue and organ damage.

- OA – obesity is common.

- Osteoporosis can occur if long term history.

- Avoid exercise in acute flare up (restrict to mobility and gentle stretching at home).

- Avoid weight bearing one week following injection.

- Avoid high impact (eg heavy chair marching) if knees or hips are involved, or if joints are unstable.

- Avoid high repetition, high strength exercises.

- Avoid overstretching; keep within the individual's natural range.

- Discontinue exercise which increases pain for more than two hours. NB Pain may not occur until the following day.

- Chronic pain and swelling may reduce performance considerably.

- Increased risk of injury.

- Ensure correct footwear and orthotics as necessary.

- Tailor to site/severity/type.

- Avoid early morning exercise.

Aims and benefits of exercise

- Improves muscle strength and power.

- Increases endurance.

- Improves bone density, balance, reaction time.

- Helps to control pain.

- Improves performance of everyday actions.

- Reduces fatigue.

- Enhances confidence and self care.

- Reduces depression.

- Improves social contact.

- Educates.

- Improves independence.

Osteoporosis

Definition

Osteoporosis is a condition in which bone mass and density gradually decreases due to loss of bone mineral, leading to loss of skeletal strength and increased risk of fracture. Common risk factors include:

- Female gender.

- Advanced age.

- Caucasian/Asian race.

- Family history.

- Low body weight.

- Early menopause.

- Prolonged amenorrhoea (cessation of periods).

- No children.

- Sedentary lifestyle.

- Smoking.

- Alcohol consumption.

- Low calcium intake.

Main characteristics

- Fractures in the spine, wrist, hip, ankle or shoulder.

- Loss of height.

- Loss of power in muscles.

- Pain.

Effects on exercise response

Exercise is likely to be limited due to fractures and bone loss affecting the shape of the vertebral column and the range of movement at the joints. There is also a likelihood of:

- Severe curvature of the upper spina (kyphosis) leading to decreased respiratory function and decreased vital capacity and problems with gait and balance.

- Limitations to the visual field leading to changes in posture.

- High risk of falls.

- Fear of falls and of exercising, leading to de-conditioning.

- Pain – either chronic or following exercise if insufficiently supported.

- Possible side effects of medication, including headaches, water retention and increase in resting blood pressure.

Pre-exercise assessment

- It is essential to establish physical limitations, spinal curvature in the upper back, balance, anxiety etc.

- Give functional tasks such as maintaining an upright posture when sitting, sit to stand, etc.

Types of exercise

- Bone loading/weight bearing/strengthening exercises.

- Target the main fractures sites – the wrists, spine and hips.

- Whole body approach.

- Mobility, stretch and postural training.

- Balance training.

- Body management, such as correct lifting technique.

- Avoid any action involving bending the spine forward.

- Avoid actions involving drawing the shoulder blades backwards against resistance, eg rowing with bands or hand weights.

- Avoid movements with any uncontrolled or unsupported trunk twisting.

- Progressive 18 month programming.

- Part of a programme with medical and nutritional supervision.

- Relaxation – physiological method to assist with stress and fatigue management.

Special considerations/cautions

- Anxiety is common, eg fear of falling and fracture. Need for reassurance and information.

- Spinal curvature alters centre of gravity, posture, gait and balance.

- Always support in standing, and in sitting when needed.

- Be aware of visual field limitations.

- Close observation and monitoring.

- Emphasise posture throughout.

- Do seated static abdominal work.

- Chronic back pain is likely.

- High levels of fatigue are likely, due to lack of fitness and poor lung capacity.

- Allow longer before progressing exercises.

- Ensure a safe working space.

Aims and benefits of exercise

- Increases muscle strength and power.

- Increases bone density.

- Reduces pain, fatigue and disability.

- Improves postural control.

- Improves balance, reaction and co-ordination.

- Improves performance of everyday actions.

- Increases confidence and self care role.

- Improves positive attitude.

- Increases social contact.

- Improves education.

- Increases independence.

Stroke

Definition

'Stroke' or cerebrovascular accident is the name given to a syndrome of rapidly developing clinical signs of local or global disturbance within the brain. This condition is caused by a sudden alteration of blood flow within the brain resulting in partial or permanent destruction of nerve tissue, leading to a wide range of functional impairments. These can include physical, sensory, cognitive, behavioural and psychological aspects.

There are two main types of stroke:

- Ischaemic (the most common) – where clots are formed due to hardening and furring of arteries.

- Haemorrhagic (less common) – bleeding from ruptured artery due to weakness in the blood vessel wall. This can be congenital, disease related, or due to injury, trauma or deformity.

Risk factors include ethnicity, raised blood pressure, the contraceptive pill, smoking, obesity, diabetes, high salt intake and lack of regular exercise.

No two strokes are exactly alike, the type of stroke, the extent of the brain damage, the part of the brain affected and the general health, fitness and attitude of the person will influence the degree of disability and overall recovery.

Main characteristics

- Paralysis or weakness (hemiparesis or hemiplegia), ie difficulties with movement and function of one side of body.

- Alteration of muscle tone – low, floppy or flaccid (hypo) or high, spastic (hyper).

- Sensory changes occur, such as diminished awareness of touch or pressure, reduced proprioception or joint position sense.

- Altered postural and balance reactions throughout the body causing difficulties with movement.

- Cognitive changes, such as deterioration in memory and planning skills.

- Perceptual changes, such as reduced body and spatial awareness.

- Visual disturbances.

- Communication difficulties.

- Depression, inability to concentrate.

- Fatigue.

Effects on exercise response

The exercise response will depend on the severity and type of neurological impairment, for example:

- High or low tone affects movement control.

- Loss of balance reactions in head, trunk or limbs causes instability in sitting, standing, walking etc.

- Sensory loss leads to impaired perception and body awareness, eg inability to identify where the leg is and execute safe movement.

- Loss of skin sensation can limit the ability to respond to pressure points, eg a saddle sore.

- Cognitive and communication disorders may limit the ability to follow instructions and give feedback.

- Most stroke survivors with a recent history of stroke are very deconditioned, due to a general lack of activity and specific movement limitations. Room for functional improvement is considerable.

- Ageing and age-related chronic disorders commonly found in elderly populations may further complicate exercise ability.

- Possible effects of medication include susceptibility to slowed responses if dose requires adjustment, and/or suppression of heart rate response

Pre-exercise assessment

It is essential to establish the effects the stroke has had on that particular person – physiologically, functionally, medically, psychologically and emotionally.

Types of exercise

- Thorough, longer warm up and warm down.

- Mobility, stretching and posture work to reduce assymetry.

- Endurance training – wherever possible, combine rhythmical, natural, low tension exercise and movement patterns with active rests. Select activities and positions where upright posture is easily achievable to reduce risk of adverse tone changes in legs or arms.

- Functional activities in standing, sitting particularly sit to stand and rocking, rolling, shuffling movements performed by moving backwards and forwards on the chair seat. Floorwork, where appropriate, is also valuable.

- Co-ordination and balance work.

- Strength training – isotonic exercise. NB avoid all strength activities that increase muscle tone abnormally or lead to abnormal associated body reactions eg shoulder lifting whilst using the arms. Avoid working to fatigue, never work to failure. Begin with a very low resistance and proceed cautiously; discontinue if there is a marked increase in tone.

- Where tone is low, ensure equipment is secured safely and comfortably. Teach how to assist the the affected side with the non-affected side to control movement. Do not hold muscle contractions for more than a slow count of three, and get participants to count out loud in order to regulate breathing.

- Relaxation – physiological method to assist with stress and fatigue management.

Special considerations/cautions

- Monitor the effect of effort on posture and tone.

- Patients are generally very de-conditioned.

- Lack of body symmetry can result in problems with gait, grip and balance. Greater care is needed in securing equipment and in controlling movement.

- There will be greater need for support and alternatives throughout.

- Heart and circulatory disease, diabetes, arthritis and frozen shoulder are all common in older stroke survivors.

Aims and benefits of exercise

- Increases quality and quantity of everyday activities.

- Decreases BP and heart rate at rest and recovery, decrease body fat regulates, blood glucose and cholesterol levels lipid regulation.

- Increases endurance.

- Increases functional strength.

- Increases speed.

- Increases co-ordination and balance.

- Increases flexibility and range of movement.

- Increases general mobility, symmetry and posture.

- Increases confidence, well being and positive attitude.

- Enhances opportunities for socialisation.

Deafness and hearing impairment

Definition

A generic term that indicates the person is hard of hearing or deaf due to partial or total loss of hearing in one or both ears. There are two major types.

Conductive deafness

This is due to a defect which prevents the conduction of sound from the external and middle ear to the internal ear, hence the person is hard of hearing. Common causes include impaction of the external ear by wax, injury or infection, and perforated eardrum.

Sensorineural or perceptive deafness

This is more serious, and is caused by interference with the inner ear's ability to process sound. Balance can also be affected because the vestibulae organs, involved in regulating balance, are also in the inner ear. Many people who are born deaf have this kind of loss. Common causes include damage to the delicate hairs or nerve fibres in the inner ear, excessive noise, infections such as meningitis, mumps, scarlet fever, measles, encephalitis or other ear infection. This type of deafness can also be caused by damage to the auditory nerve due to brain tumour.

Age-related deafness affects in one in six of all individuals aged 70 or over. All older people have a decreased ability to 'mix' sounds, screen out background noise and tolerate high pitched, high volume sounds. Tinnitus, which also increases with age, aggravates this further.

Main characteristics

- Ability to discriminate sounds decreases with intensity of sound, eg difficulty with hearing in noisy situations, for example in a group.

- Mild to moderate loss of discrimination of speech, eg decreased ability to hear TV or radio at volumes comfortable to others.

- Can lead to isolation, depression and confusion.

- Gradual onset from childhood. Up to 30 per cent loss without measurable impairment.

- May need a hearing aid.

- May experience Menière's disease – sudden attacks of vertigo, giddiness plus tinnitus, pallor, nausea and vomiting.

Effects on exercise response

- Will depend more on visual clues and observation of demonstrations.

- If following an interpreter, will be 5–10 seconds behind verbal instructions.

- Are more likely to be de-conditioned, have concentration and or relaxation problems; often appearing restless and hyperactive.

- More likely to have poorer communication skills.

- May need to wear assistive listening devices on the chest or body, behind or in the ear, or on the spectacles. Ensure these are turned on and tuned in.

Pre-exercise assessment

- Check level of hearing and whether impairment is in one or both ears, eg give a simple, audible instruction from behind the person, telling them to move their arms. Repeat it twice.

- Check if a hearing aid is worn and whether it is working properly. It should be taken out for water activities.

- Find out if an induction loop helps.

- Check if the person is able to lip read.

- If using music, check if the person can hear/feel the beat through the floor.

- Check if the person is able to use a sign language such as British Sign Language (BSL).

- Ideally show a video of what is going to take place.

Types of exercise

- As for any other participant providing they can observe and copy you.

- Postural work is often needed.

Special considerations/cautions

- Aim for effective communication.
- Ensure you can be seen.
- Use large visual cues and touch.
- Do not alter lip pattern, speak in the usual way.
- Maintain eye contact and keep mouth in view to allow for lip reading.
- Reduce background noise.
- Extra effort and sensitivity in volume and choice of music.
- Try to select venues with good acoustics.

Aims and benefits of exercise

- Improves cardiovascular fitness.
- Improves muscle strength, power and endurance.
- Improves bone density.
- Improves posture, balance and co-ordination.
- Improves range and ease of movement.
- Improves performance of everyday actions.
- Improves confidence and self esteem.
- Provides opportunities for socialisation.

Visual impairment

Definition

Visual impairment includes a range of visual perception, from partial sight to total blindness. It is the result of damage to the eye itself, or to the areas of the brain governing the interpretation of visual stimuli.

For administrative and statutory purposes, the term 'blindness' implies one of the following:

- Marked reduction of vision – less than 10 per cent in visual field (eg tunnel vision).

- Reduced visual acuity – inability to read a car number plate from three metres.

Common causes include:

- Damage to parts of the brain concerned with vision, as in birth defect, stroke, brain tumour.

- Disease or injury affecting the nerve connections between the eye and the brain.

- Major eye injury.

- Cataracts – loss of transparency of the internal lens. Can be congenital or the result of ageing or injury.

- Glaucoma – raised pressure of fluid in the eye which can cause internal damage.

- Chronic glaucoma can cause blindness if untreated. Subacute glaucoma occurs in short intermittent attacks.

- Diabetic retinopathy – damage to retina if diabetes is poorly controlled.

- Detached retina – separation of the retina from the eyeball. Vision is lost in the affected part of the retina but may be corrected surgically.

- Deficiency of vitamin A can lead to lack of retinol which can cause loss of vision in dim light and night blindness.

- Age – although an uncommon disability in childhood, blindness is a major problem in old age. Ageing affects all older people's visual acuity to some extent, peripheral vision being most affected.

Main characteristics

Physical activity is often limited and can result in:

- Poor posture.

- Obesity.

- Secondary disease(s).

Effects on exercise response

With adaptations, people with a visual impairment can participate in a range of physical activities. It should be remembered, however, that they:

- Will be unable to mirror either partially or at all.

- Have to rely on verbal descriptions and explanations.

- May require a carer or helper.

- May be performing a different movement because they cannot visualise what is expected.

- May have more balance and postural problems than other participants.

- May have difficulty in moving from one level to another, as in an exercise such as 'sit to stand'.

- Are more likely to be de-conditioned.

- May be hesitant, lacking in confidence and social skills.

- Individuals are likely to have been prescribed the spectacles or sunglasses. If they suffer from glaucoma, they will probably be taking eye drops on prescription.

- They may also be suffering from other illnesses (eg diabetes, coronary heart disease) which will affect heart rate response.

Pre-exercise assessment

- Check the type of visual impairment. Is it total or partial? Is it tunnel vision or reduced acuity (precision in peripheral vision)?

- If partial, how much can the person see or make out?

- All procedures should be verbally explored to allow the person to become more thoroughly prepared.

- Ensure the person is clear what is going to happen and agree a method of indicating all is well or some adjustment is needed. This may be verbal or tactile or both.

- Encourage rehearsal of exercises to put every one at ease.

- Encourage throughout the assessment and early stages.

Types of exercise

- Avoid impact work for people with surgically removed cataract or detached retina.

■ As for any other participant providing they can hear you and know the space.

■ Participants may prefer to do exercises on or by a chair initially.

■ If visual impairment is the secondary disease, run the programme according to needs of the primary disease with additional adaptations for visual impairment.

Special considerations/cautions

■ Ensure spectacles are secured.

■ Ensure large signs with large print. Use Braille where appropriate.

■ White cards, tape or wall markers can assist some people to orientate themselves. Highlight edges to chairs, pillars, the room etc.

■ Keep space layout and equipment the same from session to session, so that they can be memorised.

■ Tapes, handrails etc. can be useful in defining an area and accessing equipment.

■ Continuous music at the end of a space can assist in orientation.

■ Take extra care over health and safety – ie ensure there are no unnecessary objects in the working space.

■ Help in familiarising the client with the facility may be needed. An assistant or 'buddy' may be helpful.

■ Use individuals' names clearly when teaching.

■ Indicate when people arrive or leave the room.

■ Verbal instructions must be very clear and precise. Cueing must be earlier.

■ Partner activities, such as mirror work, can be effective.

■ Audiotape descriptions of the planned activity.

Aims and benefits of exercise

■ Improves cardiovascular fitness.

■ Improves muscle strength, power and endurance.

■ Improves bone density.

- Improves posture, balance and co-ordination skills.

- Improves spatial awareness.

- Improves performance of everyday actions.

- Improves stabilisation of blood glucose levels and decrease obesity.

- Improve self confidence, image and self esteem

- Provides opportunities for socialisation.

Acknowledgements

Thanks to Angie Avis, Superintendent Physiotherapist at the Joan Bicknell Centre for People with Learning Disabilities, South West London Community Trust and Helen Shilston, Community Physiotherapist and Consultant to Different Strokes, for their invaluable help and continued review of my exercise guidelines for people with specific medical conditions.

Chapter 5

Structuring an exercise session

The chair exercises in this book can be performed by most older people, from those who are completely independent and mobile to those who have limited mobility and require support from carers with daily living activities. Introducing exercise to anyone unaccustomed to activity must be done with great caution. This is even more important if the older people you are working with have chronic health conditions and disabilities, take medication or have led inactive lives for many years. We must also remember that planned exercise will be a totally new concept to most older people. It will take time for class members to learn the moves – so take it slowly and always be aware of individual differences. If participants are able, and prefer, to exercise from a standing position, most of the chair exercises can be adapted with ease. A chair back should always be provided for balance when exercises are performed standing up.

For easy referencing the exercises are described in sections to include movements for:

- Shoulders
- Chest
- Head and neck area
- Back
- Face
- Wrists, hands and fingers
- Legs and hip
- Ankles, feet and toes.

General guidelines

Table 5.1 gives a number of helpful guidelines to consider when planning activity sessions. These guidelines aim to make exercise a pleasurable, rewarding and safe experience, and so encourage individuals to make exercise a part of their daily life. Sample exercise plans are also included in the following chapter.

Frequency

If the exercises are truly going to bring benefits they must be practised regularly. Studies have shown that even low intensity exercise can bring benefits if performed frequently[1]. Just a couple of exercises once or twice a day are better than nothing. This could include a few simple upper and lower body warm up exercises followed by some slow stretching. Or decide on a weekly exercise plan and try to stick to it, say two to four times a week with sessions lasting anything from 10 to 40 minutes. Extend the programme by training an enthusiastic volunteer or 'peer' exercise leader in the class to practice short exercise routines with their fellow residents every day. This enables older people to take back some control over this particular aspect of their lives and allows the exercise group to meet in addition to regularly scheduled classes.

Intensity

If the exercises feel too easy then they are unlikely to increase fitness level. The objective is to exercise at a level just higher than the person is used to. On the other hand, exercises that feel too difficult may deter people from exercising in the future, or they may even cause distress and injury. But what is too hard? Only the exerciser is able to say how easy or difficult an exercise feels. One person may experience fatigue following just a few moments of hand clapping whilst another may be able sustain handclapping for lengthy periods. So we must constantly observe people for signs of distress and more importantly ask individuals how they feel throughout an exercise session.

Table 5.1 Exercise planning guidelines

- Individuals must choose to exercise and never be forced to do so
- Anyone experiencing illness, pain or discomfort should not exercise
- There should be a choice of exercises to suit individual abilities
- The exercises should be easy at first; introduce new exercises slowly
- Start with simple moves to warm up the muscles and joints
- The environment should be suitable for exercise (see Chapter 4)
- Individuals must 'feel safe' – eg they should have supportive chairs (see Chapter 4)
- Check recent health status of participants
- Always ask how everyone feels before, during and after a class
- Loose clothing and comfortable, low-heeled shoes should be worn
- Instructions should be friendly, informative and clear – never pushy
- Choose familiar music with a comfortable, steady beat. Ask class members for their music ideas
- Never move a person's joints or limbs for them
- Arrange for tea to be served after class and allow time for feedback

The 'talk test'

A further indication of someone's comfort level during exercise is the 'talk test', or the ability to hold a conversation during exercise. If a person is unable to talk during exercise then the exercise is too hard. The activity should never be stopped completely at this point, but a lower exercise gear must be chosen to allow the body to slow down gently. For example, if arms and legs are being exercised at the same time, the arms could be dropped and less demanding moves made on the legs and feet. Simple toe tapping would be appropriate here. Table 5.2 considers how easy or difficult an individual may rate the exercises (perceived exertion) and includes guidelines for appropriate levels of exercise to increase fitness levels safely.

There should be five segments to each class: warm up exercises with stretching, endurance activities, strengthening exercises, stretch and cool down and finally relaxation with deep breathing.

Different levels of exercise

Warm up exercises

Think of how stiff you can feel after sitting for long periods. We instinctively stretch and move slowly in order to 'wake up' the body before taking on further activity. This is also the aim of the warm up session – to prepare the body for exercise. It is an essential start to any exercise session. Light, rhythmical movements slowly increase heart rate and circulation so that muscles are warmed and joints are lubricated. Gentle stretching then completes this segment. This helps the body to respond better to exercise and more importantly, reduces the risk of muscle or joint injury.

Endurance activities

The endurance section is commonly called aerobics. Activities which make the heart and lungs work harder, such as running and walking require some degree of aerobic training. The ability to do such activities means we have ample reserve capacity to continue to cope comfortably with daily living activities such as housework, running for a bus, shopping, gardening and self care. An older frail person who has been inactive for a very long time may have virtually no reserve capacity available for even the simplest, basic everyday living activities. Without steps to reverse this decline the inevitable outcome is total dependency.

Where older people are unable to walk or run, chair exercises can mimic these actions. For example, slow marching with corresponding arm work will make extra demands on the heart and lungs so they can become stronger and more efficient in providing blood and oxygen to all parts of the body.

Strengthening exercises

General muscle strengthening plays an essential part to achieving good all round physical condition. Resistance training using weights or resistance bands can make the muscles and bones stronger and increase joint stability.

However, weights and resistance bands should be introduced carefully and slowly. Initially, strengthening exercises that use only the person's own body weight to move arms and legs may be sufficient to produce positive changes, especially in the frail older person who has been inactive for many years. Apply the talk test often to help understand how much effort is being spent. As participants progress, light weights or resistance bands can be added so that the programme remains challenging. I prefer to use resistance bands for strength training.

Exercises 50 to 55 illustrate how to include these bands in your activity sessions.

Stretch and cool down exercises

This section of the programme allows heart and breathing rates to return slowly to normal. Many of the exercises used in the warm up and endurance sections can be repeated at a much slower pace for the cool down period. Since the muscles, joints and ligaments have been warmed from previous activity, this is a good time to include more gentle stretching to tone and lengthen the muscles surrounding the joints. Hold the stretches for 6 to 10 seconds to encourage suppleness. To increase flexibility, gradually add longer stretches of up to 20 seconds – but never over stretch. Stretching must always feel comfortable.

Table 5.2 Perceived exertion chart

1 Comfortable, able to talk naturally
2 Comfortable, starting to feel warm
3 Feeling warm and comfortable – able to talk easily
4 Breathing a little harder, able to talk easily
5 Feeling warm and a little 'puffed' – able to talk comfortably
6 Continues to feel 'puffed' but still breathing regularly and able to hold a conversation comfortably
7 Feeling much warmer, working harder to perform moves, can still comfortably maintain a conversation
8 Feeling very warm, finding moves harder, unable to hold a continuous conversation
9 Out of breath and very tired; unable to talk or perform the exercises properly
10 Feeling 'over puffed', hot and exhausted

Relaxation with deep breathing

Deep breathing and relaxation can help to reduce the negative effects of stress and tension and encourage self-awareness by promoting positive feelings. Chapter 8 covers this subject in more detail.

- Aim at level 1–3 for the warm up and cool down period

- Aim at level 3–7 for the endurance exercises

- Return to level 2 or 3 before moving on to another part of the programme

- As fitness increases aim at higher levels – but never aim past level 7

- Exercises must never feel painful

- Participants must be able to pass the 'talk test' whilst exercising

Adapted from the Borg Perceived Exertion Scales[2].

Exercise guide

Many of the exercises in this book are clearly illustrated and all have step by step explanations on how to perform the moves. Safety tips are included and each exercise also clearly indicates (see abbreviations below) which part of the exercise programme is under consideration.

WU	=	warm up
E	=	endurance
ST	=	strength training
S	=	stretching
CD	=	cool down

For example, shoulder shrugs (Exercise No.1) is an effective warm up and cool down (WU, CD) move for the shoulders and neck area. You will notice that many exercises can be adapted for use in several segments. For example, the slow march (Exercise No. 32) can be used in the warm up, endurance and cool down (WU, E, CD) segments. In this case – the slow march in the endurance section would be performed a little faster than in the warm up and cool down sections.

Start by first going through the exercises yourself and then again with a friend. Repeat the exercises again, this time working to music that has a strong, rhythmical beat. Try the exercises from a standing position and compare how they feel to exercising from a sitting position. Imagine how you would manage the exercises if one side of your body was affected by weakness or paralysis.

The beginners' programme

Start with a short light programme to include one or two exercises from the warm up (WU), cool down (CD), breathing and relaxation segments. The exercises are performed slowly with good posture and regular breathing. Increase the selection of exercises gradually, remember that some individuals expend great effort to continue even the simplest exercises if they have been inactive for long periods. Once everyone feels comfortable with such a beginners' programme, add a few stretches (S), endurance exercises (E) and strengthening (ST) moves.

Progression

Progress by increasing the time spent exercising and by raising the level of difficulty –

but always gradually to allow people to learn and perform the moves correctly. For example, spend a few minutes longer on the warm up by repeating slow head to toe movements. Follow this with a few stretches to prepare the areas you plan to use in the endurance section – such as feet and arms. Extend the endurance section by a few minutes too if everyone is comfortable.

Try stringing exercises together, for example, the stretch and fist exercise (No. 23) may be followed by the piano playing exercise (No. 24) which would neatly lead on to the conductor's baton (No. 28). Add some of your own ideas to the programme – such as circling the hands and wrists. Keep the circles small to start with and gradually make these larger, again watching for good control. Click or point the fingers, clap hands on the thighs, then clap hands together at chest level, taking the hands down towards the floor and upwards above the head. Add the arms, using a strong rowing or swimming action. Also use the feet to link the exercises, for example, slow marching, alternate foot tapping, 'can can' kicks etc. As balance and coordination develop, try exercising hands and feet together, always starting with the most simple moves, such as toe taps and hand clapping. Further progression is achieved by adding more exercise repetitions (see page 93) and also by exaggerating the moves so they are larger, but always well controlled.

The strengthening exercises can be made more demanding with the introduction of resistance bands (Exercises 50–55). The timing for this depends entirely on individual progression.

The exercises

Starting position and posture check – all exercises will start from these positions unless otherwise stated.

Chair exercises:

- Check that the chair is fully supporting the back, bottom and thighs.
- Those with good balance may prefer to sit slightly forward in the chair (but should not lean forward).
- Keep the back and neck as straight as possible.
- Think about trying to lift the chest as though preparing to take a deep breath.
- Arms should be close to the side of the body, with the hands comfortably by the side or in the lap.
- Muscles should be tightened but not over tense (the knuckles should not be white, any equipment used should not be gripped too tightly, jaws should not be clenched).
- Feet should be flat on the floor, the legs should be one hip width apart for good balance.
- Knees should be over the toes with the knees and toes pointing forward.
- Breathing should be regular, natural, not held.
- If feet do not touch the floor, a book or foot rest may be used to support the feet.
- Use a chair raise if legs are too long and the seat height too low.

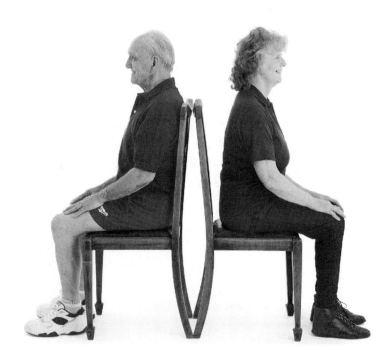

For exercises performed standing

- Always have a sturdy, high backed chair available to hold onto for balance.
- Feet should be planted firmly on the floor a hip width apart to give a secure base.
- Knees are slightly flexed, never rigid and straight.
- Pelvis area should be tucked in a little and stomach muscles pulled in comfortably.
- Keep the back as straight as possible, but not rigid.
- Shoulders should be away from the ears, and arms held comfortably by the side.
- The neck should be lengthened, with the chin parallel to the floor and the eyes facing forward.
- Normal breathing should be maintained throughout.

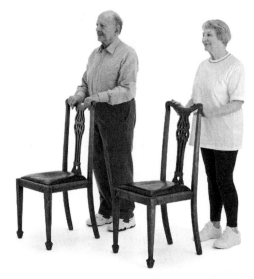

For exercises performed in bed

- The head and neck should be supported with a pillow.
- Arms should rest comfortably next to the body, with the shoulders relaxed.
- Body should be lengthened.
- Legs should be straight, but the knees relaxed.
- Kneecaps and toes should be pointing upwards.
- A small, folded towel may be placed in the small of the back and under the knees for extra support.

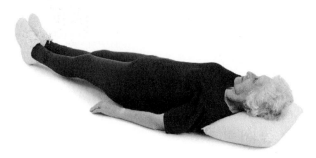

Shoulder and arm exercises

Many of these moves are perfect for the warm up period to prepare the muscles and joints for further exercise. I particularly like these exercises as participants often shuffle their whole body around in order to move their shoulders. These simple moves also help to get rid of the stress and tension we all seem to readily store in our neck and shoulders. Always start with small moves, arms held quite close to the body.

■ Progress with larger moves away from the body.
■ Check starting position and posture and review safety tips.
■ Aims – to ease tension in the shoulders and gently warm these joints.

1 Shoulder shrugs (WU,CD)

This move can also be done whilst in bed with arms at the side.

1 Slowly lift both shoulders to a shrug.
2 Hold the shoulders for just a moment.
3 Release the shoulders and allow them to drop down, pulling them down a little further than normal.
4 Gently release the shoulders and they will find their natural position.

Repeat four times.

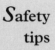

Safety tips

● Always start slowly and keep the movements fluid, not jerky.

● Try not to allow the head to drop forward because this may arch and strain the back.

● If doing this exercise in bed, keep the legs relaxed. The knees may be slightly bent if this feels comfortable.

● A small folded towel placed in the small of the back may increase support and comfort.

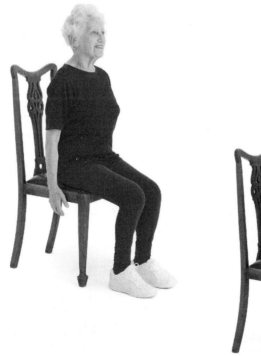
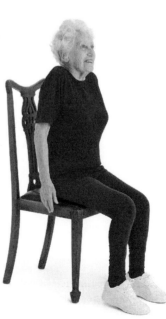

2 Shoulder rolls (WU, CD)

1 Raise the shoulders.
2 Then gently roll them forwards in a circular motion.
3 Push them back.
4 Return to the starting position.
5 Repeat – rolling the shoulders backwards this time.

Repeat four times.

3 Swinging Shoulders (WIJ, CD)

1 Lean slightly forwards.
2 Take the opposite arm and lower it over the edge of the chair.
3 Allow this arm to move forwards and backwards, parallel to the body.
4 Keep the arm relaxed but at the same time do not allow the arm to swing out of control.
5 Swing the arm in small circles, forwards and backwards.
6 Repeat this exercise with the other arm, taking plenty of time to get into position.

Both arms can also be exercised together if balance is good.

Repeat four times.

4 Front crawl or doggy paddle (WU, E, CD)

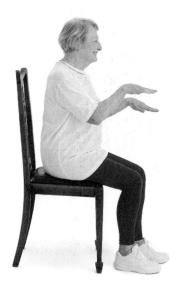
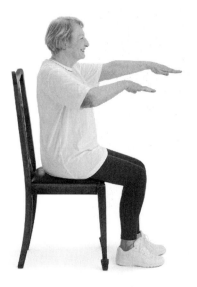

1 Start with the arms close to the chest.
2 Reach forward slowly with one arm, and then back, as if pulling forward through water.
3 Repeat with the other arm and continue in a rhythmic swimming action.

Repeat four times.

Progress by taking the arms further away from the body and by making the moves larger.

5   Backstroke (WU, E, CD) and back of arm stretch (S)

For the backstroke:

1   Sit tall with knees slightly apart and directly over the ankles.
2   Hands should be on the lap or by the side.
3   Raise one arm up and over the head as if brushing the hair.
4   Return arm to starting position and repeat with the other arm.

For the stretch:

1   Raise one arm again (slowly) over the head.
2   Then lower the hand and rest it on top of the head.
3   Slowly slide the hand down the back of the head to touch the back of the neck.
4   The elbow should be pointing upwards and the palm facing inwards.
5   Hold the stretch for a few seconds and then return the arm slowly to the starting position.
6   Repeat with the other side.

As flexibility improves, it may be possible to reach further down the back with the hand.

Repeat four times.

Safety tips

- Raise the arm only to a level that is comfortable – even if this means the arm must remain to the front of the body.

- Support the stretching arm with the free hand if required.

- As flexibility improves, progress by taking the arm to the back of the head and by also increasing the reach down the back.

- Keep the arm close to the body.

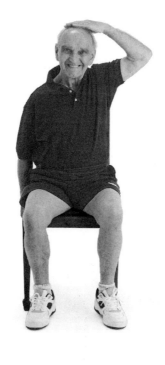

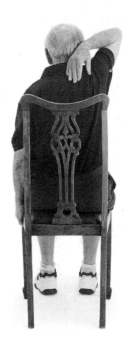

6　Breast stroke (WU, E, S,CD)

1　Place hands together, at chest level, as if praying.
2　Allow hands to drop forward so fingers are pointing straight in front.
3　Push arms slowly out in front of chest, stretching arms and fingers.
4　Take arms out to side and back to starting position.

Repeat four times.

7　Arm and shoulder stretch (S)

1　Stretch both arms out towards the knees.
2　Lightly rest the hands on the knees – fingers together and pointing outwards.
3　Maintain the stretch and then slowly raise arms to chest level.
4　Hold the stretch here for a moment before continuing to raise the arms above the head if this feels comfortable.
5　Hold for a couple of seconds, then lower the arms to chest level and finally back to the starting position.

Repeat four times.

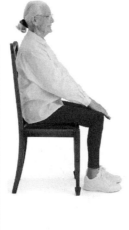
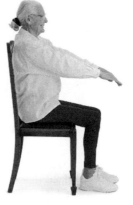
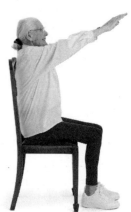

8   Chair push ups (ST)

This is a strengthening exercise for the shoulders, but it also makes demands on arms, hands, back, thighs, knees and feet. Another very important benefit is that this can relieve pressure on the sacral area. A full standing position may not be the aim or be possible for everyone. In this case, even moving into position for this move (without actually standing or rising from the seat) is a worthwhile target.

1   Place hands firmly on arm rests or at the edge of the seat next to the thighs.
2   Bring feet slightly back towards the chair and place them firmly on the floor at hip width.
3   Sit towards the front of the chair, stomach muscles are pulled firmly in.
4   Without bending or tipping head forward, push off with arms and legs to lift the bottom out of the chair.
5   Continue in an upward movement to the standing position if possible.
6   Slowly return to a sitting position, keeping the head held high and leading into the chair with the bottom.

This exercise may also be carried out in bed. Raise the knees, push the feet and arms into the mattress to raise the bottom slightly off the bed.

Repeat several times throughout the day.

Safety tips

● It is important to rise from the chair in an upward movement, keeping the back as straight as possible to avoid falling forward.

● Many class members will be unable to raise themselves out of the chair. Do not force this move – just getting the body into the ready position for this move will initially be quite enough for some.

● Those with loss of function on one side can press down with the unaffected side to correct posture and sit as tall as possible.

● Breathe normally throughout the move.

● Prepare for this move with warm up exercises for the feet and legs.

● This move needs to be supervised initially.

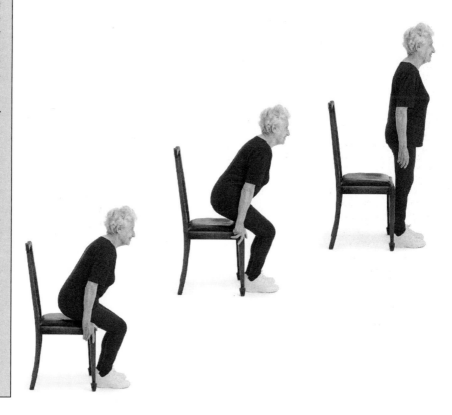

Chest muscles

These exercises are designed to build upper body strength by strengthening the chest and upper back muscles. Both these exercises can be done whilst in bed.

Check the starting position and posture. Review safety tips.

9　Palm press (ST)

1　Press palms together in front of the chest.
2　Hold for a few seconds, then relax and repeat.

10 Shoulder pull (ST)

1　Lock the fingers in front of the chest and pull in opposite directions.
2　Hold for a few seconds and then relax and repeat.

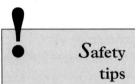

Safety tips

- Breathe normally throughout.
- Keep finger locks quite loose to avoid strain on finger joints.

Head and neck exercises

All of us have suffered from stiff necks at one time or the other. Those who fall asleep in their chairs throughout the day tell me they often wake up with a stiff jaw and neck. These simple movements can be done anywhere and at any time to help ease stiffness and promote good posture in the head and neck area. After all, who wants a pain in the neck?

Aims – To ease tension and maintain or increase mobility in the base of the neck (cervical joints).

Check starting position and posture before each exercise.

11 Head turns (WU, S, CD)

1　Start with head raised in a natural, forward-facing position.
2　Keeping to shoulders still and facing forwards, gently turn head to one side and hold for a few moments.
3　Gently return the head to the starting position.
4　Then very gently turn the head into the other direction and hold for a few moments
5　Slowly return the head to the starting position.

Repeat four times.

Safety tips

- These moves are very small and very slow – please also see safety tips at the end of this section

12 Head press (ST)

1 Using the previous starting position, bring one hand up and place the ball of the palm on the forehead.
2 Gently increase pressure from the hand onto the forehead.
3 At the same time, press down onto the hand with the head.
4 Maintain the pressure on the head and hand, then release.
5 The head should not be moving in any direction.

Repeat four times..

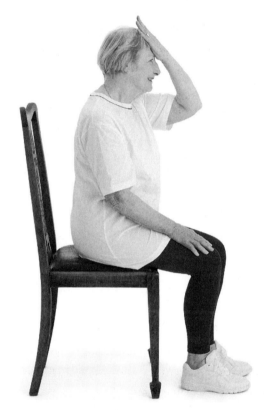

13 Chin pull (S)

1 Hands should be on the thighs.
2 The head should be held comfortably level, facing forwards.
3 Pull the chin towards the chest as if to make a double chin (the chin is pulled in and not tipped down).
4 Slowly return the head to the starting position.

Repeat four times.

Back exercises

Many of the older people I see in care spend lengthy periods sitting in a chair. This can put a great deal of pressure on the spine and surrounding muscles which can in turn become overworked and fatigued.

A healthy back is a strong back. Strong back muscles keep the spine erect by helping to protect the integrity of the spinal column. This promotes good posture and the ability to move with balance and confidence. Bad posture means that the spinal column, muscles and ligaments are under a lot of abnormal stress. A hunched back also puts pressure on the chest and abdominal organs. Lungs may not be able to expand fully, and the digestive system may be compromised. The back may also be further weakened by diseases such as osteoporosis and arthritis.

Other muscle groups come into play when we use our backs. Hip, leg and stomach muscles need to be strong so they can share the workload placed on the spine. It is in this way they can support and prevent injury to the spine.

These simple exercises concentrate on good posture. Difficult moves, such as bending forward at the waist without support, are avoided as these can overly strain an already weakened back.

Check starting position and posture. Review safety tips.

Aims – To help to relieve stiffness in the spine, tone surrounding muscles and encourage good posture.

14 Back press (ST)

1 Place hands on the knees or chair arms (without gripping hands tightly).
2 The bottom is placed well back in the chair.
3 Lean back into the chair – feel the chair back supporting the spine.
4 Stomach muscles are pulled in, the feet and thighs help to push the spine back.
5 Hold the head up, looking straight ahead (never tilt the head backwards).
6 Hold the spine firmly into the chair for a couple of seconds.
7 Slowly release the back from the chair.
8 Relax the thigh and stomach muscles but maintain good posture.

Repeat four times.

15 Trunk twist (S)

Being able to twist and turn confidently means that individuals can turn to talk to a neighbour, look out of a window or help themselves to objects nearby without falling over.

1 Use the starting position and check posture.
2 Place the left hand on the right knee or right chair arm.
3 The right hand rests gently on the right hip.
4 With the hips quite still and facing forward, gently turn the head so it looks over the right shoulder.
5 Gently pull in the stomach muscles.
6 Hold this position for four seconds, feeling a comfortable twist in the spine.
7 Slowly return the head and shoulders to the front.
8 Remove the left hand from the knee or chair arm.
9 Remove the right hand from the hip.
10 Maintain good posture and take a deep breath before repeating this move on the other side.

These exercises can also be performed in bed with supervision. Just make certain that the knees and toes point upwards, and the knees remain soft (not locked). Use a small pillow to support the head and neck.

Repeat this four times.

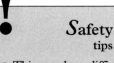

Safety tips

- This may be a difficult move for some people. Reduce the twist by adjusting the hands so that they both rest on the thigh (instead of one hand on the hip and the other hand on the thigh).

- The head should be turned slightly to one side.

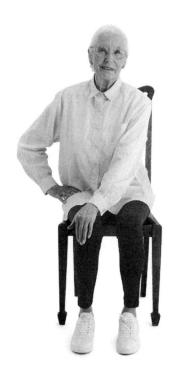

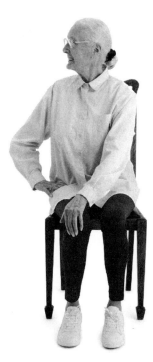

Safety

tips

- Never lean forward from the hips without support.

- Never try to force or complete exercises which feel uncomfortable or painful.

- If any exercise causes pain in the legs or hips, it must be discontinued.

- Perform each exercise slowly, the various stages should flow into each other without any jerky moves.

- Those with stomach or spinal problems should refrain from these exercises. Specialised consultation with a physiotherapist or doctor may be required to find appropriate alternative moves for those with such complaints.

- Breathe normally throughout the moves.

16 Sitting arch (S)

This is another simple move to relieve stiffness in the shoulders, neck and back.

1 In the starting position, the bottom should be firmly back in the chair.
2 Place hands on knees or lightly hold chair arms for support.
3 Slowly drop the head to look at the knees.
4 Follow with the shoulders curling gently forwards, followed by the spine.
5 Do not lean forwards – the back should remain firmly against the chair.
6 The stomach should be pulled in firmly.
7 Hold this position for four seconds.
8 Gently release, starting from the spine, working the way up to the shoulders and last of all the neck and head.

Repeat four times.

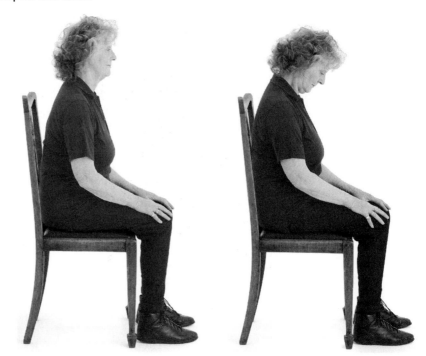

17 Upward stretch (S)

Perform this move in the chair or on the bed (with legs lightly flexed). This move helps to relieve stiffness in the back and shoulders and reinforces the good posture position.

1 In the starting position, the feet should be firmly planted on the floor.
2 Place the left hand on the chair seat by the left thigh or rest the hand in the lap.
3 Raise the right arm out in front to chest level.
4 The head should be level and facing forward.

5 Bring the raised arm in and rest the hand on top of the head.

6 Now turn the elbow out so that it presses towards the chair back.

7 Release the tension and then raise the arm above the head.

8 Hold for a couple of seconds before lowering the arm and placing the hand back on the head.

9 Rest the arm here for a couple more seconds before lowering the arm back onto the lap.

10 Rest for a moment, maintaining good posture.

11 Repeat with the other side.

Repeat four times.

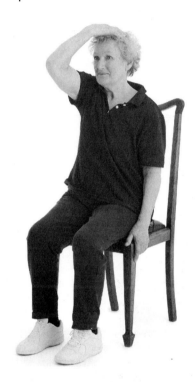

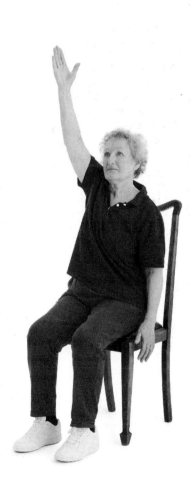

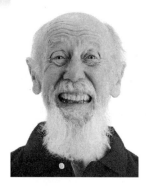

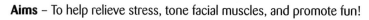

Facial exercises

Maybe we don't laugh enough? The need to laugh is as basic as the need for love, security and faith. It has been said that we don't stop laughing because we get old, we get old because we stop laughing. A hearty chuckle is a wonderful way to tone facial muscles, ease tension in the jaw, shake off the blues and lift the spirits. Laughter also has a wider effect, it stimulates heart muscle activity, increases circulation and oxygen intake. Heart rate then decreases following laughter, muscles are more relaxed and tension is eased.

These light hearted exercises can be done anywhere and at anytime. They will be good for stressed out carers too!

Aims – To help relieve stress, tone facial muscles, and promote fun!

Check starting position and posture. Review safety tips.

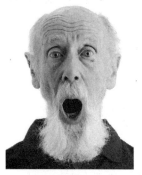

18 Tongue loosener (WU, CD)

1 Head and shoulders should be relaxed.
2 Hands should be relaxed and resting on the lap.
3 Slightly open the mouth.
4 Lift the tongue and gently press it to the roof of the mouth.
5 Hold that position for four seconds.
6 Release the tongue and allow it to fall back into its natural position.

Repeat four times

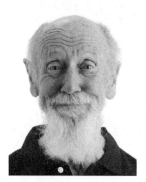

19 Vocal vowels (WU, CD)

This will help to loosen the jaw and exercise muscles around the mouth.

1 If possible, place two fingertips over each jaw hinge (just below the ear lobes) to feel the jaw move throughout the exercise.
2 Say aloud the first vowel 'A' using an exaggerated expression.
3 Repeat this with all five vowels.
4 Completely relax hands and jaw in between each set of exercises.

Repeat four times

We often use colloquial sounds in our classes here in Yorkshire – such as 'Eee Bah Gum!' We try to exaggerate our pronunciation and usually end up in a fit of giggles. So have a go at tailoring this exercise to your particular region.

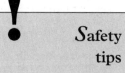

!

Safety tips

● Only open the jaw within comfortable limits. The jaw area is easily dislocated so NEVER over extend the jaw

20 Forehead frown (WU, S, CD)

The forehead is another area prone to stress.

1 The head should be comfortably balanced on the neck with the eyes looking ahead.
2 Open the eyes widely, feeling the pull on the forehead muscles.
3 Hold this position for two seconds.
4 Slowly allow eyes to relax.
5 Then close the eyes gently and continue to close until they are firmly closed.
6 Once again, feel the tension in the forehead and the muscles tightening around the eyes.
7 Hold this position for two seconds.
8 Gently release the squeeze until eyes are opened and relaxed.

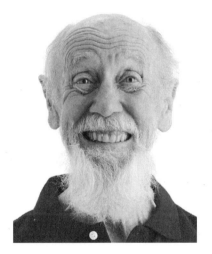 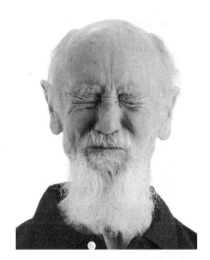

Wrist, hand and finger exercises

Normally our wrists, hands and fingers are constantly being exercised as we go about our daily work. This opportunity may be reduced or even totally removed if everything is done for us. Whilst accepting the fact that many of us may require some help with difficult manoeuvres at certain times in our lives, we must remember that if joints are not regularly used they will become weak, stiff, unstable, and prone to contracture deformities.

The important message here then is to encourage movement through daily living activities. For example, washing through 'smalls', handkerchiefs etc in the bathroom sink, dusting, helping in the kitchen, pursuing handcrafts and playing games such as dominoes, cards or skittles. Regular, planned exercise is also an easy and effective way to maintain or even improve range of movement.

In this section we look at simple exercise routines that carefully move and stretch the joints through their full range of movement. A couple of tennis balls will be required for the last exercise in this section. Specialist product companies (see the Resources section) can supply very useful hand exercisers, such as exercise putty, at reasonable cost.

Most of these exercises can be done anywhere and ideally they should be carried out several times a day if possible. Bath time is an excellent opportunity for such exercises. Alternatively, place the hands in a bowl of warm water. Movement is easier when joints are supported by water, and the warmth of the water also adds a soothing and beneficial dimension.

So let us start with some moves to warm up the fingers and wrists, using one or both hands at the same time. Never force these moves through pain or discomfort, although gentle movements can help maintain mobility. A gentle stretch is what we are aiming for. The doctor may need to assess any problems and with the help of other health professionals, such as physiotherapists, give advice about the correct balance of rest and exercise.

Hand and finger exercises

Hands may be raised in the air or supported on the lap, bed or table.

Check starting position and posture. Review safety tips.

Aims – To help preserve fine finger movement, increase circulation to extremities, discourage stiffness and contracture.

21 Finger spread (WU, ST, S,CD)

1 With the elbows tucked in, rest hands on a firm surface or raise hands to chest level and point fingers ahead.
2 Slowly spread the fingers widely apart.
3 Hold for a few moments.
4 Slowly close fingers.

Repeat four times.

22 Finger lifts (WU, S, ST)

1 Rest both hands on a firm surface.
2 Start by lifting the thumb off the surface.
3 Hold for a few seconds before slowly returning the thumb to its starting position.
4 Then repeat each finger, one by one.

Repeat two times.

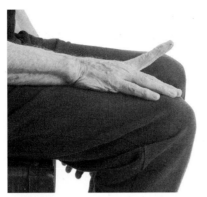 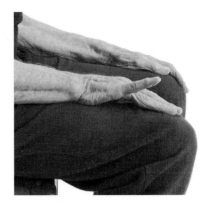

Finger lifts

23 Stretch and Fist (WU, S,CD)

1 Keeping the arms close to the chest, lift hands (palms down) and point fingers in front.
2 Maintain a comfortable stretch for a few seconds.
3 Then gradually curl the fingers into a loose fist.
4 Repeat two times.
5 Return to the position described at 1 above, and repeat this exercise with palms facing upwards this time.

Repeat four times.

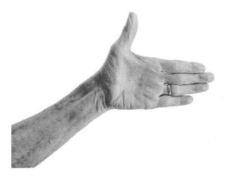 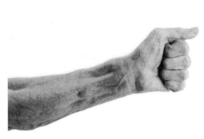

24 Piano playing (WU, E, CD)

We have lots of fun with this move, building up a rhythm for a very effective endurance exercise. Start with small moves initially; progress with larger, stronger, higher, and lower actions which make the whole body move and sway. Add some of your own moves to make a routine. This may include hand clapping, hand circling, shaking hands (as if trying to get them dry), for example.

1 Point the fingers out and 'wiggle' them as if playing the piano.
2 Move the hands from side to side as if playing piano scales.
3 Try changing direction – wiggle the fingers up and down and side to side.

Repeat four times.

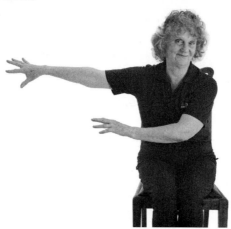

25 Fingers to thumb (WU, S, ST)

1 Raise one hand slightly, or rest the heel of the hand on the lap with fingers raised.
2 Bend the index finger so that the tip meets the tip of the thumb on the same hand.
3 Hold this position, gently pressing these tips together.
4 Keep the other fingers as straight as possible.
5 Slowly release and straighten the index finger.
6 Repeat this process with all the other fingers, one at a time, keeping other fingers as straight as possible.
7 Once all the fingers have been exercised in this way, repeat the process starting from the little finger.

Repeat two times.

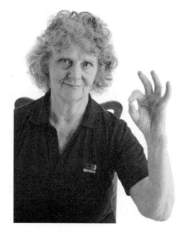

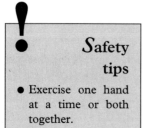

!

*S*afety
tips
● Exercise one hand at a time or both together.

Safety tips

- Exercises can be performed with one hand at a time.
- The full finger stretch must never be forced, especially where there are joint deformities.
- Never exercise painful or inflamed joints.
- Keep fists loose to avoid joint strain.

26 Finger press ups (WU, S, ST)

1 Put the palms together in a praying position or, if only using one hand, use a firm surface.
2 Press the fingertips on one hand firmly against other hand.
3 Slowly move the palms out and away from each other, keeping fingertips firmly together.
4 Hold this position and slowly increase the pressure on the fingertips.
5 Slowly return to the starting position.

Repeat four times.

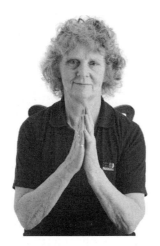
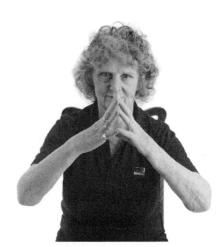

Wrist exercises

These exercises can be carried out virtually anywhere at any time. Exercise both wrists together or one at a time.

Aims – To maintain or increase strength and flexibility in the wrists.

27 Forward flap (WU, S, ST)

1 If supporting the hands on a surface, place hands at the edge so that fingers can drop down.
2 Start with hands and fingers gently stretched out in front.
3 Raise hands as if ready to push away.
4 Hold for a few moments keeping the arms as still as possible.
5 Slowly lower the hands; continue to allow them to drop below the level of the wrist until a comfortable stretch is felt.
6 Maintain this hold for a few seconds.
7 Then return slowly to the starting position.

Repeat four times.

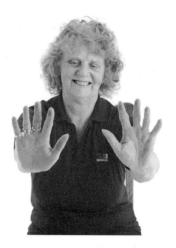
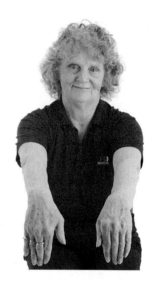

28 Conductor's baton (WU, E, CD)

Everyone is transported to the last night of the Proms with this one when we play 'Land of Hope and Glory' and 'Rule Britannia' on the tape deck. We swing our make believe batons and imagine we're conducting the orchestra and choir. Once again, start with slow moves (use softer slower music in the warm up and cool down segments). Then make the moves larger and stronger for the endurance section.

1 The hands should be in a loose fist – as if holding a baton.
2 Raise the hands to chest level, initially keeping the arms quite close to the body.
3 The action is from the wrist. Make the shape of a triangle in the air like a conductor who is leading his orchestra.
4 Make the horizontal move first, then take the wrist upwards (to the upper point of the triangle) and then bring the arm down to the point you started from.

Repeat four times.

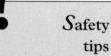

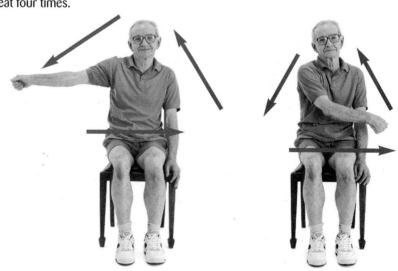

29 Wrist pushover (WU, S, ST, CD)

1 Raise hands and place together as if praying. The elbows should be out to the side and close to the chest.
2 Press hands firmly against each other.
3 Push hands slowly over to one side and hold for a few moments.
4 Return to the starting position.

Repeat four times.

30 Wrist lift and press (ST)

1 Place hands on a firm table.
2 Press firmly down on surface with flat hands.
3 Hold for a few seconds.
4 Release the pressure and repeat.
5 Place hands underneath table and press with palms upwards, as if trying to lift the table.
6 Hold for a few seconds before releasing the press and repeat.
7 If a table is not available, press down on lap or bed to achieve the press and use one hand against the other for the lift.

Repeat four times.

31 Wrist and grip strengthener (ST)

1 Using one hand at a time can make it easier to concentrate on the exercise, but two hands can be used if desired.
2 Keep the elbows close to the body.
3 Arms can rest comfortably in lap.
4 Hold the tennis ball in palms that are facing upwards with fingers comfortably spread.
5 Squeeze the ball firmly, slowly increasing pressure on the ball and hold for four seconds.
6 Keep the wrists straight (avoid bending hands inwards).
7 Breathe normally throughout.
8 Slowly release the grip on the ball.

Repeat four times.

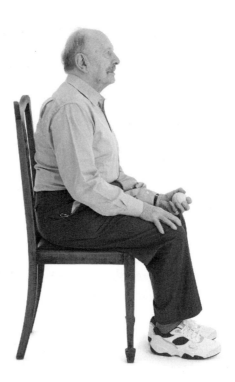

Legs and hip exercises

Strong thigh and leg muscles are needed for walking. Even when the older person is not mobile, strong thighs help when they are transferring from bed to chair, chair to bath etc. Strong legs also help to maintain good posture whilst sitting. Walking and stair climbing probably offer one of the best ways to maintain limb strength and must be encouraged wherever possible. When these activities cannot be carried out, chair exercises can contribute to balance, and to maintaining sufficient flexibility for simply moving around in the chair so that, the person can turn to speak to a neighbour or look out of a window.

Knees are major weight-bearing joints and, as such, are subject to a high degree of stress and strain throughout our lives. They are also a common target for inflammatory conditions such as rheumatoid arthritis. During acute arthritic episodes the knee joints can become painful and swollen making movement difficult. This is not the time for exercise. Joints should be rested, assessed and treated by the physiotherapist or doctor. Gentle exercise may be possible once the acute pain and swelling subside.

Increasing inactivity, arthritic disease, osteoporosis and past hip injuries may all contribute to stiff and weak hips. Hip exercises may also involve movement of the spine and so prove beneficial in this area too. Choose chair, water or bed for almost any of these moves.

Many of the exercises below can be performed while the person is in the bath when joints and muscles are warm. The water provides soothing comfort and support, but the moves must be performed slowly and never forced.

Check starting position and posture. Review safety tips.

Aims – To take the knee joints through their own normal movements to maintain or increase function, flexibility and strength. To practice normal hip movements, reduce stiffness and increase suppleness in these joints.

A few simple toe taps and heel raises will help to warm up the legs in preparation for the following exercises.

32 Slow (on the spot) march (WU, E, CD)

1 If needed, hold loosely on to the side or arms of the chair for extra stability.
2 Slowly lift the right knee upwards, with the toes pointing downwards.
3 Hold this position for two seconds.
4 Slowly lower the foot keeping good control all the way down.
5 The toes should touch the floor first, rolling onto the ball of the foot, followed by the heel.
6 Rest for a couple of seconds before repeating with the left knee.

Repeat four times.

33 Knee bends (WU, CD)

1 If needed, hold lightly on to the chair seat edge for balance.
2 Lift the right leg, bend the knee and take the foot back towards the chair, keeping the weight on the toes and ball of foot.
3 Do not force the foot under the chair. The toes should be level with the front chair legs.
4 Hold for two seconds before slowly resuming to the starting position.
5 Rest for a couple of seconds before repeating with the left leg.

Repeat four times.

34 Leg extension (ST)

This and the following exercises also exercise the hips.

1 Once again, hold lightly onto a chair for extra security.
2 Gently lift the right leg out in front and straighten the leg (do not lock the leg).
3 Hold for two seconds.
4 Slowly lower the right leg and return it to the starting position.
5 Repeat with the left leg.

Repeat four times.

Safety tips

- Never force these movements.
- Keep the moves very small to start with.
- Knees must point forwards all the time, twisting can lead to serious injury.
- When straightening the legs, never lock the knees.
- The non-exercising foot must be placed firmly on the floor.
- Breathe normally throughout.

35 Knee bends in bed (ST)

This exercise provides very simple moves to perform in bed.

1 Lay flat on the bed with a pillow to support the head and neck.
2 Slowly bend one leg up and hold for a few seconds (rest the foot on the bed if the leg feels too heavy).
3 Stretch the leg back out to the starting position.
4 Repeat with the other leg.

Repeat four times.

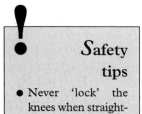

Safety tips

- Never 'lock' the knees when straightening legs.

- Avoid dragging the foot on the bed.

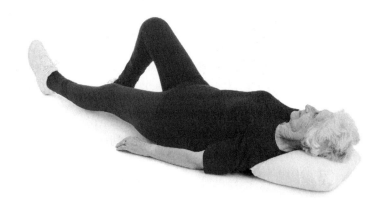

36 Leg lifts in bed (ST)

This exercise follows on from the bed knee bends.

1 Start from the flat position with toes pointing upwards.
2 Slowly raise one leg slightly off the bed and hold for two seconds.
3 Lower the leg back onto the bed and relax.

Repeat four times.

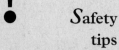

Safety tips

- Avoid throwing the leg out; keep all moves under control.

- Never exercise swollen, painful or inflamed joints.

- Start with very small moves.

- Take rest periods in the beginning and check posture again at these times.

37 Leg kicks (WU, E, CD)

1 Check for good posture.
2 For extra support, gently hold on to the edge of the chair seat.
3 Raise the right leg and gently take the leg out in a slow, well controlled kick.
4 Return the leg to the starting position, landing on the toes and ball of the foot.
5 Repeat with the left foot.

Repeat four times.

38 Tennis ball thigh squeeze (ST)

1 The hands should be on the lap or by the side.
2 Thighs and knees should be together.
3 Place a tennis ball between the thighs.
4 Gently squeeze the thighs together to hold the tennis ball firmly in place.
5 Hold for a couple of moments, then release.

Repeat four times.

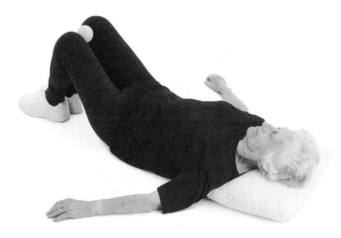

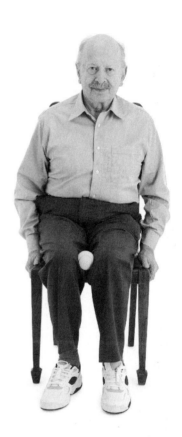

> **!**
>
> ### Safety tips
>
> ● Hold on to the side or front of the bed for balance if required but avoid gripping the bed too tightly.
>
> ● Keep legs straight and knees 'soft' if performing this move in bed.
>
> ● Breathe normally throughout the move.
>
> ● Toes and knees should always face the same direction.

39 Sit to stand (ST)

This exercise is similar to the Chair push up exercise (No.8), but the Sit to stand exercise concentrates on using thigh strength to reach a standing position, rather than using the shoulders and arms. For those with mobility problems standing may not be possible. In this case, the exercise can be practised in stages – even moving into position for the exercise takes some effort and is a worthwhile goal.

1 Sit towards the front of the chair, pulling the stomach muscles in firmly.
2 Bring feet slightly back towards the chair and place them firmly on the floor at hip width.

3 Keep the back long, and lean forwards slightly without bending or tipping the head forward

4 The hands should be firmly but lightly on the thighs. Feel the thighs and legs take the weight in preparation to stand.

5 Rise out of the chair in an upward movement, breathing normally.

6 Stand as tall as possible, then prepare to return to the chair.

7 Hands should be lightly on thighs. Keep a good upwards posture and lower the body into the chair, leading with the bottom.

Repeat several times a day.

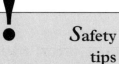

Safety tips

- There is often the temptation to lean forwards, supervision and assistance with balance is necessary until there is good posture and control.

- Please see safety tips for Exercise No.8.

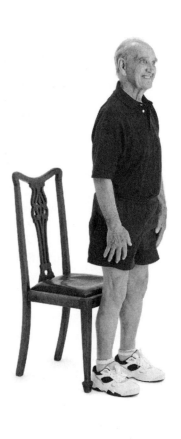

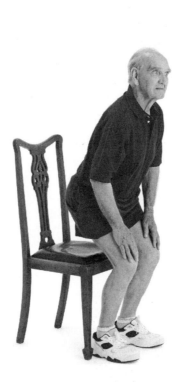

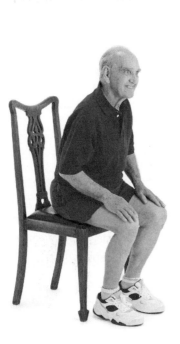

40 Hip circles (WU, CD)

Keep these moves very small to begin with.

1 From the starting position, with legs on hip width apart and knees over the toes.
2 Gently raise the right leg just a few inches off the ground.
3 Make a small circle using the whole leg, working from the hip.
4 Rest for a couple of seconds before circling in the other direction.
5 Repeat with the other leg.

Repeat four times.

41 Tropicana wiggle (WU, ST, CD)

This exercise gives an opportunity to play Salsa music and keep the beat with castanets or maracas (see also exercise No. 49). It can be performed very slowly to ease pressure from sacral areas, as a strengthening exercise for the legs and hips or slightly faster as part of a movement to music routine.

1 Lightly hold onto chair edge or arms, feet are firmly planted on the floor (or bed) for good balance.
2 Push off from the right foot so that the body sways slightly to the left side and the right hip is almost raised from the seat.
3 Hold for two seconds.
4 Return to the starting position.
5 Repeat with the other side.

Progress to 'walking' to the front of the chair and then 'walking' to the back of the chair.

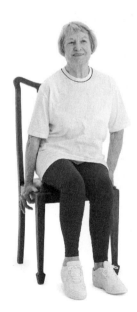

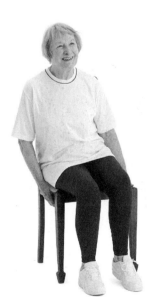

Ankle, feet and toe exercises

Healthy functioning feet and legs are necessary if any level of mobilisation is the goal. Movement can also strengthen the joints, tendons and ligaments making feet less susceptible to sprain or injury. Studies have shown that many falls suffered by older people occur when muscle mass loss results in ankle weakness[3]. Falls are the leading cause of accidents in the elderly. They are also a major source of hospital and nursing home admissions[4].

But before we consider exercises for the feet, it is essential to understand the importance of supportive footwear for standing and walking. Soft, fluffy bedroom slippers may be comfortable, but they offer little support and encourage the wearer to shuffle along instead of walking heel to toe. Shoes with good support increase confidence and balance, a vital consideration if mobility is to be a genuine target. One solution might be to keep a pair of supportive shoes nearby (in a locker or even under a chair) so these can be easily slipped on as required throughout the day.

These exercises are also useful following prolonged periods of sitting, especially to 'wake up' the legs and feet before standing or walking.

Check starting position and posture. Review safety tips.

Aims – To increase or maintain flexibility and strength in the ankles, feet and toes.

42 Toe Curls (WU, S, ST, CD)

This is a good exercise to do whilst still in bed. One foot at a time may be used if preferred.

1 Make certain feet are quite flat on the floor or supported on the bed.
2 Concentrate on feet and slowly curl the toes under.
3 Hold the curl for a few seconds.
4 Slowly uncurl, stretch and separate toes.
5 Allow toes to fall back into their natural position.

Repeat four times.

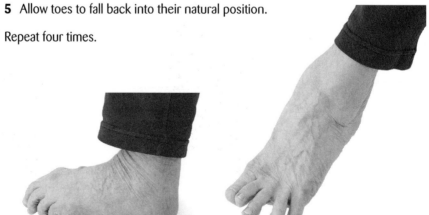

Safety tips

- Raise toe and heels gently until a comfortable stretch is felt.

- Never force a stretch – ligaments and tendons may be stiff and the range of movement limited.

- Bones in the heels can be delicate. Always place the heel down on the floor gently to avoid injury.

43 Heel Raise (WU, S, ST, CD)

This move can be added on to Exercise 42 in various combinations. For example, you could try a heel raise following each toe tap or heel raise following right and left toe taps.

1 Feet should be flat on the floor to start with.
2 Keeping one foot on the floor, raise the other heel and let the ball of the foot take the weight.
3 Maintain the hold for a few seconds.
4 As the heel slowly returns to the floor the other heel is gently raised in the air.
5 Continue raising heels alternately.

Repeat four times.

44 Rocking feet (WIJ, ST, CD)

Flexion in the ankles also involves the calf muscles which act as a pump to assist the return of blood from the lower limbs, thereby encouraging increased general circulation. Once again start with one foot at a time and progress to both feet.

1 Feet should be flat on the floor, to start with.
2 Raise toes off the floor, taking the weight gradually on the heels.
3 Hold for a couple of seconds.
4 Return the toes to the floor.
5 Once the toes touch the floor, slowly raise the heels off the floor, taking the weight on the ball of the feet.
6 Repeat again, aiming for a controlled flowing movement from heels to toes.

Repeat four times.

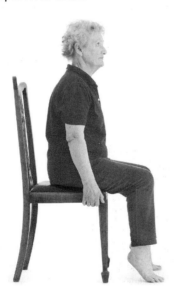
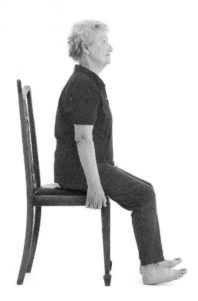

45 Foot circles (WU, S, ST, CD)

Wake up tired feet with this one – anywhere! It is good for the aching feet of health care workers too!

1 Work one foot at a time.
2 Raise one foot just clear of the floor.
3 Gently circle the foot in one direction.
4 Change directions and circle the foot again.
5 Slowly replace the foot on the floor.

Repeat four times with each foot.

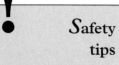

Safety tips

● This exercise is best avoided by those suffering from painful, arthritic joints.

● Start with very small moves to warm up muscles and ligaments.

● Knees should be facing forward and quite still throughout this exercise.

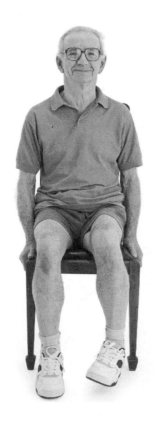
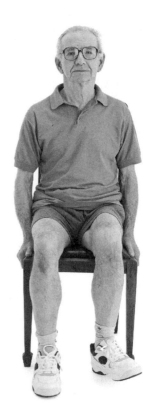

46 Toe taps (WU, E, CD)

Music with a strong rhythmic beat gets just about everyone's toes tapping.

1 Start again with feet flat on the floor.
2 Slowly raise the toes of one foot, keeping the heels firmly on the floor.
3 As toes return to the floor, the toes on the other foot are raised.
4 Continue this alternate toe tapping.

Repeat throughout the exercise session, keeping the moves small and controlled.

47 Toes in, toes out (ST)

1 Start with feet flat on the floor – a hip width apart.
2 Raise the toes off the ground and lightly turn on the heel until the foot is pointing slightly outwards.
3 Lower the toes.
4 Raise the toes again, lightly taking the weight on the heels, and return the feet to the starting position.
5 Lower the toes.
6 Raise the toes, turning lightly on the heels towards the middle.
7 Lower the toes.
8 Raise the toes once more and return the feet to the starting position.

Repeat four times with each foot.

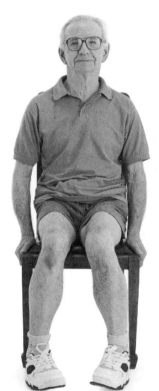
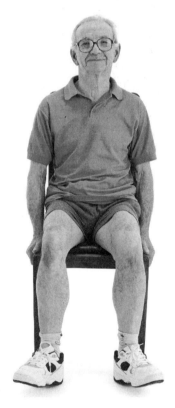

Safety tips

- Aim for very small moves from the ankles.

- The knees and toes must always face the same direction.

- Take the weight lightly on the heels; don't dig them into the floor.

- Twisting actions are not recommended for those with arthritis or joint problems.

- Exercise one foot at a time if preferred.

Safety tips

- Always start with small steps, heel to toe.

- Discourage shuffling, gently lift and place the whole foot on the floor if heel to toe flexion is difficult.

48 Three steps out – three steps back (WU, E, CD)

Encourage a heel to toe movement walking out, reverse this on the way back.

1 Take a small step with the right foot away from the chair.
2 Follow with the left foot and once again with the right foot.
3 Bring the right foot back one small step.
4 Do the same with the left foot.

5 Take another step back with the right foot.

6 Both feet should now be level and comfortably placed under the knees.

Repeat four times.

49 Basic salsa step (WU, E, CD)

Find some upbeat Latin American music and have some fun with this one. Maracas or castanets add to the fun and help to keep the rhythm.

1 Start with both feet flat on the floor.

2 Move the right foot back towards the chair so the right toes are level with the left heel.

3 Working with the beat of the music, return the right foot to its starting position.

4 Repeat with the left foot.

Repeat four times.

Adding resistance to exercise

These are advanced exercises for older people who have participated in regular exercise over a period of time. There is no specific time to introduce weights or resistance bands. It depends entirely on how each individual progresses through earlier exercise routines Some people may find the exercises becoming very easy after a few weeks, and may therefore feel ready to add a little extra difficulty to some of the moves. Others may take many months to get to this level. Exercise programmes must continue to be challenging or the muscles will adapt to the same old exercise. Adding weight or resistance to a programme can supply this challenge and help to reduce frailty, poor mobility and fatigue by increasing muscle tissue, bone strength and general circulation. It also increases motivation by adding new interest.

Resistance bands

I prefer to use elastic bands to add resistance to the exercises. Always make certain individuals are fully warmed up before moving on to this section to avoid injury. The bands are especially made for resistance exercise and` come in various strengths. They can be bought from sport shops or ordered from catalogues (see the Resources section). Start with the lightest strength.

Making a start

Add a few minutes of strength training into existing exercise programmes, increasing this segment as individuals adapt to the changes. Perform the exercises without resistance bands until everyone can perform the moves correctly. It is wise to strength train just two or three days a week to allow the muscles a recovery period. It is possible to strength train more often, but only if large muscle groups are

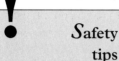

Safety tips

● Start slowly to warm up the ankles and feet.

● Maintain good control over each move. Work very slowly to begin with so each step is executed with good control.

● Keep the feet light.

● Add the arm work for only short periods at first and keep arms at chest level.

rotated. For example, the upper body could be exercised on Monday and Thursday and the chest and lower body exercised on Tuesday and Friday.

Participants will find these exercises easier to perform in chairs without arms. However, some individuals with balance problems feel unsafe without the added security of chair arm supports. In these cases, exercises should be performed with arms inside the chair. Firm foot rests may be required for those in wheelchairs.

Those using resistance bands for the first time may notice it takes quite a bit of effort to stretch the bands. Consequently they may be tempted to hold their breath as they make the effort to stretch the band. Breath holding can place abnormal strains and demands on the heart, causing a sharp increase in blood pressure. Breathing should be regular, breathing in through the nose during the easiest part of the move and out through the mouth during the hardest part. A further way to discourage breath holding is to simply hold a conversation with people during exercise. It is very hard to hold your breath when you are talking.

Progression

The exercises will get easier when they are practised regularly. Increasing the number of exercises (repetitions) will keep the programming challenging and effective. For example, the exercises below are to be repeated four times to start with. Progress by repeating this set (of four) exercises once the individual feels stronger and ready for an extra challenge. This means the exercise is repeated four times, with a short pause before repeating the exercise four times again. Further progression is added by increasing the number of exercises (repetitions) in a set. For example, repeat the exercise five times instead of four times. Continue increasing the number of exercises performed in one set until a maximum of ten moves are performed in one go. Progression is directly related to each individual's capabilities and it may take several weeks or months to build up to sets of ten.

Keep a record of each person's weekly sessions and progress. This can help to plan safe progressive exercise and allow the person who is exercising to see just how much they are accomplishing.

Starting position for strength training

1 Good posture, with the bottom well back into the chair, back and neck as straight as possible, supported by the chair.
2 Those with good balance may prefer to sit slightly forward in the chair (but should not lean forward).
3 The backs of the legs should resting against the chair seat.
4 Feet should be planted firmly on the floor, hip width apart for balance.
5 Keep the resistance bands as wide as possible and hold firmly without over-clenching the fist.

*E*xercise Safety tips

1 Never hold the breath during exercise.

2 Apply the 'talk test' regularly to gauge effort.

3 The moves should be rhythmical, never jerky.

4 Keep arm movements low at first to prevent shoulder strain.

5 Keep the wrist rigid and the elbow slightly flexed to prevent tendon and ligament injury.

6 Wrap the band widely around the forearm when there is any arthritis or tenderness in the hand or wrist.

7 Never hold one position (static) for more than five or six seconds.

8 Hold movements over the head for no longer than two or three seconds.

9 Muscles may feel comfortably tired following exercise but never painful.

Aims of strength training – To improve general fitness and increase the ability to perform everyday activities.

Check starting position and posture. Review safety tips (see Chapter 4).

*S*afety tips

- Try to keep the grip on the band fairly light to avoid too much tension on finger joints.

- For those with a weak grip, wrap the band around the hand a few times. This will reduce the need to grip the band so tightly.

- The band may also be secured under the hip. Sit on the band if the hand is not strong enough to take the strain (see exercise step 2 above).

- Slacken the band if it is too difficult to stretch.

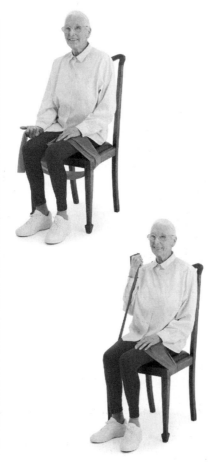

50 Front arm curl

This exercise strengthens the upper arm muscles (biceps).

1 Place the resistance band underneath the chair and hold on to each end of the band.

2 Now place the left end of the band onto the left hip and hold down securely with the left hand (as shown).

3 The other end of the band is held firmly in the right hand, palm facing upwards.

4 Keep the left upper arm close to the body.

5 Slowly raise the lower part of the left arm at the elbow so that the band is stretched towards the right shoulder.

6 Keep the upper arm and shoulder quite still during the move.

7 Pause and then return the left arm to its starting position.

8 Repeat with the left arm.

Repeat four times.

51 Back arm curls

This exercise strengthens muscles behind the upper arms (triceps).

Check starting position and posture.

1 Secure one side of the band on the hip or under the thigh.
2 The photograph shows how the band is then taken around the back of the chair.
3 The other arm is taken over the head and then bent behind the head so the hand is behind the neck.
4 The elbow points upwards and the hand firmly grasps the free end of the band (palm facing inwards).
5 Extend this arm slowly upwards above the head – the band is now stretched comfortably.
6 Then slowly return the hand to the back of the neck.
7 Check for good posture and then repeat, taking the arm upwards and downwards, always in a controlled manner.

For an alternative way to secure the band – tie the resistance band to the back of the chair or the exercise instructor can hold the band behind the chair.

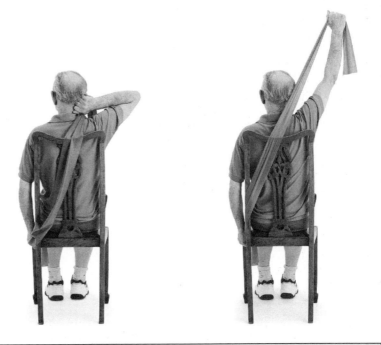

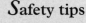

!

Safety tips

- Watch for good posture – avoid arching the back during the lift.
- Breathe normally throughout.

52 Front arm raise

This strengthens the front of shoulders.

Check starting position and posture.

1 Place the resistance band underneath the chair and hold on to each end.
2 Hold each end of the band with palms facing inwards (as though hands are on a steering wheel).
3 Slowly stretch the band out in front, until the arms are parallel to the floor.
4 Pause and then slowly return the arms to the starting position.

Repeat four times.

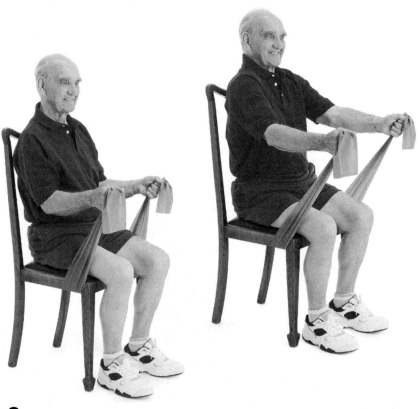

Safety tips

• Never lock the arms when extending them outwards.

• Remember to breathe out during the hardest part of the exercise.

• One arm at a time may be exercised. Secure the other end of the band under the opposite hip or have someone hold the other end of the band.

53 Side arm raise

This strengthens the upper back and shoulders.

Check starting position and posture.

1 Once again, place the resistance band underneath the chair and hold on to each end.
2 Feet are a hip width apart.
3 Hold firmly on to each end of the band with palms facing inwards (in the same position as for the previous move).
4 Take the arms out to the sides, away from the body.
5 Keep the arms straight but do not lock the elbows.
6 Raise the arms to a comfortable position, aiming to raise the arms no higher than shoulder level.
7 Pause before slowly resuming to the starting position.

Repeat four times.

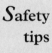

Safety tips

- Do not lock the elbows.

- This can be quite a difficult move as the arms are held away from the body – keep the band quite loose to start with and only lift the band to a comfortable level.

- One arm may be exercised at a time. Follow the safety tips as for previous exercises.

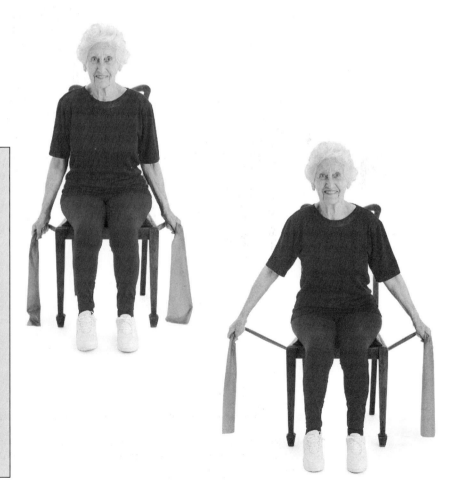

54 Leg extensions

This exercise strengthens the muscle at the front of the thigh.

Check starting position and posture.

1 Place the centre of the band under the right foot.
2 Hold the ends of the band in both hands, rest hands on lap.
3 Raise the right foot in front until is the leg is quite straight but not locked.
4 Pause before returning to the starting position.
5 Repeat with the left leg.

Repeat four times.

!

Safety tips

● If hands are not strong enough to hold bands, or if there is only one hand available, tie the two ends of the band together and place the knot over the thigh. The foot is then placed in the lower part of this sling. The tied end can then be held down easily with one hand, or the instructor could help to secure this knotted end onto the person's lap.

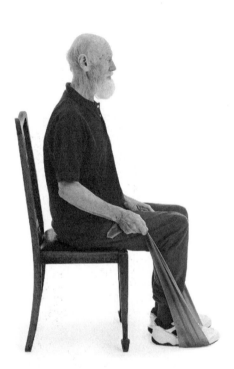

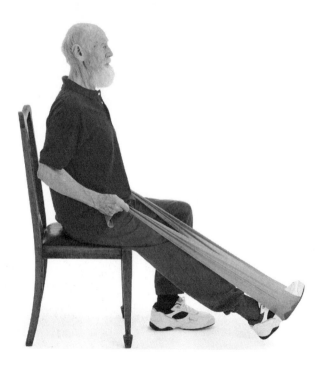

55 Hip abductors

These strengthen hip muscles and help to prevent joint stiffness.

Check starting position and posture.

1 Place the resistance band underneath one foot.
2 Secure the ends of the band by the side of the other hip, arms are close to the body.
3 The non-exercising leg is a hip width away from the other leg and the foot is planted firmly on the floor.
4 Slowly take the exercising leg a few inches out to the side.
5 Pause before slowly returning the leg to the starting position.
6 Pause once more before repeating the exercise.

Repeat four times.

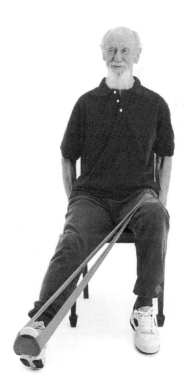

Safety tips

● See tips for the previous exercises.

● Those with hip injuries or problems may need to seek specialised consultation with a physiotherapist or doctor before trying this exercise.

References

1   Shephard, R.J. (1990) Exercise for the frail elderly. *Sports Training, Medicine and Rehabilitation,* Volume 1, pp: 263–277.

2   Borg, G. (1970) Perceived exertion as an indicator of somatic stress. *Scandinavian Journal of Rehabilitation Medicine*, No. 293, pp:92–98.

3   Van Norman, K.A. (1995) *Exercise Programming for Older Adults.* Human Kinetics, Champagne, Illinois.

4   Skelton, D. (1998) Prevention of falls. *Research into Ageing News.* 9 (Summer).

Chapter 6

*D*aily living activities

If we are aiming for good all-round physical condition then we must encourage a balanced mix of activities. Structured exercise is not the only way to increase activity. An excellent way to keep fit is to use existing habits and build activity into the daily routine. Normally we are involved in a wide range of activities as we go about our daily jobs, responsibilities, hobbies, housework etc. Although we do not generally tend to think of these activities as exercise, they nevertheless contribute to our overall fitness. There is also evidence to suggest that residents lead happier, healthier lives if they are encouraged to take more responsibility for their own care.[1]

Including activity in daily routines

Traditionally, helping people in supported settings has concentrated mainly on doing things for residents, such as grooming, dressing, feeding, lifting and so on. While many older people require such attention in times of illness and disability, completely taking over these daily living activities can seriously undermine self care, discourage everyday activities and promote increasing dependency. We, as health care workers, also lose the opportunity for genuine participation in the rehabilitation of people who trust us to do the very best for them.

As carers we have a responsibility to change our perception about what helping older people really means. Sometimes it is quicker to take over an older person's personal care completely. However, this saves time in the short term only. In fact no time at all is saved if carers must do everything for everybody, every day. Supporting, instead of taking over an older person's daily living activities, will admittedly require a little extra time at first. However, in the long term everyone benefits if residents can increase their strength, flexibility, balance and confidence and so assume increasing responsibility over their own daily living activities.

Many older people seem to just give in and allow things to be done for them. For example, Marion would always allow her carers to take her whole weight during transfer from wheelchair to armchair instead of herself trying to make some effort. When older individuals are given no encouragement to do things for themselves, their lives become increasingly controlled by others and the motivation to help themselves in any way is lost. In Marion's case, simple encouragement and commands, as shown below, have made a positive difference and although she is unable to move from one chair to another on her own, she is now making the effort to use her legs and feet during transfer.

We would start by explaining to Marion what was going to happen and how she could help:

'Marion, we are going to help you move from this wheelchair to your armchair.'

'Take your feet off the foot rests and place them firmly on the floor – feet a little apart (hip width) for good balance.'

'Now move slightly forwards in the chair – we will keep the chair steady for you.'

'Push down on the chair arms with your hands and feel your feet and legs take the weight as you prepare to stand, we will help you to keep your balance.'

'Think about keeping your legs strong as you stand and try to keep your head up and your back as straight possible.'

'Now take small steps towards the chair until you feel the chair seat touching the back of your legs.'

'Hold onto the chair arms and slowly lower yourself into the chair seat – bottom first.'

'Take a moment and then place your hands on the chair arms and your feet firmly on the floor so you can lift yourself further back into the seat.'

'Is this is a comfortable position for you?'

'That worked very well Marion. We will try to take a few more steps the next time.'

Carers and nurses are in a prime position to help residents increase their activities through the specific care they deliver throughout the day. This is also a very good way to get to know individual capabilities before progressing with a group exercise session. Another important advantage is the reduced risk from over exertion as activities are spread throughout the day instead of being concentrated into one exercise session.

Here are some suggestions of how to include activity into care routines:

Wake up stretches

These simple moves are carried out in bed. They provide a good way to wake up the body and prepare for the day ahead.

- Slow stretching from top to toe – keep the arms and legs quite straight against the body.

- Stretch fingers and toes, relax and stretch again. Circle the hands and wrists, one way and then the other.

- Raise shoulders towards the neck (as if shrugging the shoulders) and slowly release. Repeat several times.

- Then slowly raise the arms above the head and stretch the fingers before returning arms to the bed.

- Raise just one arm this time and take it over the body so the fingers touch the opposite shoulder.

- Repeat with the other arm, then return arms to side of body.

- Bring one knee up towards the body – stop at a comfortable position and rest the foot flat on the bed.

- Then bring the other knee up to join the first knee.

- Feet are now firmly on the bed, push down on the bed with the arms and hands (palms down) and try to raise the hips off the bed.

- Hold for a few moments and then return hips slowly to the bed.

- Keep one leg bent with foot flat on the bed – straighten out the other leg (but do not lock the kneecap). Slowly raise the straight leg a few inches off the bed.

- Hold this leg in the air for a few seconds and slowly rotate the ankle one way and then the other way (keeping the kneecap quite still throughout the move) before slowly returning the leg to the bed.

- Repeat this with the other leg.

- Raise the right leg off the bed a few inches once again (keeping the other leg bent at the knee with the foot flat on the bed) and this time move the straightened leg slowly outwards just a few inches.

- Return the leg to the centre and then slowly lower the leg until it is resting on the bed.

- Repeat with the left leg.

- Return to the starting position and allow the body and mind to relax completely for a few minutes.

- Maintain regular, normal breathing throughout all the moves.

Personal care

Exaggerate moves used in washing, cleaning teeth, combing hair, dressing, and so on. There may be many opportunities to move the arms forwards and upwards during the day, but very few daily activities take the arms upwards and over the head. Shoulders grow stiff and muscles at the back of the arm (triceps) atrophy and weaken. So simple care activities, such as combing hair, become progressively difficult or even impossible.

Older people with a weak grip or arthritic hands may find it difficult to hold a brush or comb adequately. If this is the case, the handle can easily be built up to facilitate grip by using tape or bandage. Many other everyday items may also be adapted for safe and easy use: examples include utensils, pen and pencils, zips and buttons on clothes, water taps, medicine bottle tops, to mention but a few. Occupational therapists, physiotherapists and specific product brochures (see Resources section) can offer further help and advice with specialised aids that make life easier for people with disabilities or restricted mobility.

Initially, the more frail individual may not have sufficient power or flexibility to take the comb or brush back towards the head. Never move the person's arm for them – only a suitably qualified practitioner such as a physiotherapist can do this safely. Use large, slow movements to demonstrate the full range of movement and encourage the individual to copy the action to the point where they remain comfortable and in control of their actions. In time, and with regular practice, the range of movement may be extended so that some or all of this aspect of personal care can be returned to the person.

It is well worth considering some of the other problems that may affect an older person's ability to increase activity and self care. For example, poor hearing and eyesight can affect confidence, balance, depth perception and coordination. These problems can often be overlooked or simply accepted as inevitable. Older people themselves often fail to report problems because they 'don't want to bother the doctor'. Whilst some of these problems may be difficult to relieve, others may have relatively simple solutions that can revolutionise an older person's life. For example, a number of older people accumulate large amounts of ear wax which can cause or compound deafness. In some cases, ear syringing can often provide almost instant relief. Of course ear syringing must always be performed by trained nurses following a doctor's examination. Many people also

wear hearing aids and these need to be checked regularly to ensure they are working efficiently. An eyesight examination may uncover the need for a new prescription lens or sight may be improved by simply cleaning a foggy pair of spectacle lenses.

Bath time

The warmth of the water creates the perfect environment for moving and stretching the body. Movement is also easier when joints are supported by water. Push the normal actions of bathing a little further than normal, for example, take the bath sponge and reach over to the opposite shoulder, stretch to touch the knees, ankles and toes, reach behind the head to wash the hair, neck and shoulder areas. The wake up stretches (bed exercises) recommended earlier can easily be adapted for use in the bath. Those with painful or inflamed finger joints may also benefit from a little extra time to exercise hands and fingers in the warm, soothing water.

Toileting

Another opportunity to encourage residents to try the chair push up exercise (No.8) with the aim of increasing control over their muscles when transferring over to the toilet. Older people who rely totally on others for their toileting needs have told me this is the activity they wish they could regain control of more than anything else.

Some people also suffer from additional problems such as urinary incontinence, but this should never be accepted as an inevitable consequence of ageing. There are several types of incontinence and any such problems should always be referred to a doctor so conditions such as constipation and urine infection, which can cause or increase incontinence, can be ruled out or treated. Other specially trained health professionals such as district nurses and continence advisors can also help to alleviate or make incontinence less stressful.

Pelvic floor exercises

Sometimes exercises can help if incontinence is caused or aggravated by weak pelvic floor muscles. These are the muscles that line the floor of the pelvis and give support to the pelvic organs and their outlets. A weak pelvic floor muscle can cause the bladder to leak. Just like any other muscle in the body, the pelvic floor muscle will get stronger if it is exercised regularly. These exercises can be performed when standing, sitting or lying down – Table 6.1 shows how to do these exercises from a sitting position.

Table 6.1 Pelvic floor exercises

- Sit comfortably in a chair with legs relaxed and slightly apart
- Imagine you are trying to stop yourself from passing wind from the bowel, but try not to clench the buttocks
- Feel the back passage tighten and lift away from the chair
- Now imagine you are also trying to stop passing urine
- Again feel the urine passage lifting away from the chair
- Practice this exercise several times a day

Meal times

A good opportunity to perform fine finger movements and practice coordination skills. Whilst some residents may be unable to cut up their own food and always require help to do this, others may be able to take some control over their own food plate if simple interventions are used. For example, a non-slip mat placed under the plate will stop the plate moving away. Utensil handles may need building up or specially made cutlery may be available for those who are unable to grasp a regular knife and fork. A water jug on a tipping cradle may allow residents to pour their own drinks. A comfortable, secure position at the dining table is also important, the person who is unable to reach the table adequately will lose some of the power required to cut and organise their meal.

Preparing for sleep

Help to induce a pleasant sleepy feeling with slow stretches (in bed) combined with the relaxation and deep breathing techniques described in Chapter 8.

Social activities

In the care home setting, a programme of social events can be a wonderful way to increase activity, revive old hobbies, learn new skills, develop friendships and share fun times with the staff. A well thought-out programme includes something for everyone, such as bingo, dominoes, music appreciation, sing-a-long, craft making, quiz games, slide shows, and local outings. The activities are suggested by the residents, who also help to plan and supervise the activities. If the home you are working in has no social activity programme, then start your own. Ask residents which activities they would enjoy participating in and create an events diary to plan and coordinate these ideas. Begin with simple activities such as bingo, skittles, poetry recitals and sing-a-longs. Involve the residents in all the stages of planning and ask colleagues for their ideas and contributions. Managers and matrons are usually very keen to support these programmes. Those placing their older relatives in care also need to know that their loved ones are being cared for in a rich, stimulating environment.

Finally, just a few other ideas I have seen used in care homes to increase activities and promote a higher quality of life.

- Pets – many homes have a resident budgie, cat or dog. Residents enjoy stroking, talking to, caring for and having fun with these pets.

- Invite residents to help at meal times with tasks such as buttering bread, laying trays and tables, making pastries and collecting cups and saucers.

- Gardening – raised flowerbeds and adapted gardening tools make it possible for some residents to enjoy light gardening work. Or why not bring some of the outside inside with houseplants or herb boxes? Residents often enjoy growing and tending to plants in their own rooms.

- Spring cleaning day – where residents do as much housework in their rooms as possible, from light dusting to vacuuming.

- Even literary talents can surface when residents are asked to contribute to a newsletter. Such contributions could include poetry, art, news articles, humorous pieces, crosswords or an events diary for example.

Reference

1   Jones, R.A. (1985) *Research Methods in the Social and Behavioral Sciences*. Sinauer Association Inc., Massachusetts.

Chapter 7

Sample exercise plans

The following plans are provided as a guide to give you an idea of what a typical exercise session looks like for beginners (levels 1 and 2) and for those with more experience or ability (levels 3 to 5).

Start slowly with simple moves so that each person has plenty of time to learn and perform the moves correctly. Always include a good selection of exercises for all levels of abilities. Avoid any twisting moves or moves that suddenly change direction, and always emphasise good form and posture. Remember, it may take several weeks before some older people are ready to progress with longer sessions or more difficult moves.

Structuring a typical exercise plan

A one-to-one exercise session is the perfect place to start. As the instructor you can focus your attention on just one person, and this person will also enjoy the individual attention. Talk to the person you are working with, ask him or her what feels good and what is difficult. Take all this feedback into consideration when structuring future classes.

Level 1 – Exercises in bed

Try starting with exercises in bed. Use the wake up stretches as described in Chapter 5. This gentle stretching routine can help the older person to face the day in a positive way. All the moves are very small and must feel comfortable. This routine can also be repeated when the person retires to bed for the night. Add a few minutes of relaxation and deep breathing (see Chapter 8) to help induce tiredness.

With practice this routine will become very easy and you may wish to suggest including a few strengthening moves into the morning routine (keeping the evening routine simple and calm). Gradually add the following moves to the morning routine – repeat each exercise 2–4 times initially.

Finger spread (Exercise No. 21)

Finger lifts (No. 22)

Fingers to thumb (No. 25)

Finger press ups (No. 26)

Palm press (No. 9)

Wrist pushover (No. 29)

Shoulder pull (No. 10)

Tennis ball thigh squeeze (No. 38)

Toe curls (No. 42)

Bed push up (No. 8)

Remember, it may not be possible for the person to execute the moves fully. Older people who have led sedentary lifestyles, or have perhaps been dealing with chronic illness are likely to have a narrowed range of motion. With time and practice the person's range of movement will grow. *Never* force the movements.

Level 2 – Beginners' chair activities

This includes simple warm up and cool down moves for those who may be new to exercise and/or have been sedentary for lengthy periods. The moves are selected to promote flexibility and range of movement. Choose motivating music with a strong, slow beat and always pay close attention to posture and form. Discuss the particular benefits of each exercise, for example shoulder shrugs and shoulder rolls to reduce

stiffness and keep the joints in good working order for dressing and undressing. Also allow plenty of time to explain and demonstrate how to perform the moves correctly.

Shoulder shrugs (Exercise No. 1)

Shoulder rolls (No. 2)

Swinging shoulders (No. 3)

Head turns (No. 11)

Tongue loosener (No. 18)

Vocal vowels (No. 19)

Forehead frown (No. 20)

Doggy paddle (No. 4)

Breast stroke (No. 6)

Finger spread (No. 21)

Stretch and fist (No. 23)

Piano playing (No. 24)

Slow march (No. 32)

Toe curls (No. 42)

Heel raise (No. 43)

Foot circles (No. 45)

Toe taps (No. 46)

Complete the session with the wake up stretches (as used in Level 1), relaxation and deep breathing.

Level 3 – Adding progression to chair activities

Repeat Level 2 but this time create a little rhythm to the session by linking the exercises to each other. Simple clapping and foot tapping between the exercises maintains the flow and gives everyone time to prepare for the next move. Maintain a very slow pace throughout, gradually increasing the pace (for endurance) when everyone is ready to do so. Continue with a long, slow cool down. Finally, add a few simple stretches, for example :

Arm and shoulder stretch (Exercise No. 7)

Stretch and fist (No. 23)

Forward (wrist) flap (No. 27)

Toe curls (No. 42)

Foot circles (No. 45)

As always, end each class with relaxation and deep breathing.

Level 4 – Progress the routines

You can progress by adding a little difficulty and variety into the routines. Vary the exercise combinations with other exercises in this book and increase the number of repetitions. Too many exercises can confuse everyone – including the instructor! So keep it simple and introduce new exercises slowly to help people learn and remember the moves.

In Level 3, we linked exercises with hand clapping and foot tapping. Now add some of your own ideas to keep the session flowing, for example hand shaking, hand circles, small arm circles etc. For the feet, in addition to simple toe tapping, try slow marching and small leg kicks to link the moves. To further challenge the muscles and stimulate the mind I often include a 'round robin' in my classes. This is where I invite everyone in turn to lead the class for a few minutes.

Further progression is made by moving the arms and legs together, as if walking with slow marching (Exercise No. 32) and swinging shoulders (No. 3). Gradually make the moves larger. For example, doggy paddle (No. 4) is initially performed with small hand and arm movements near the chest. These hand and arm movements can be made larger (but always with good control) and the arms taken further away from the body, also in different directions, high and low and side to side. This means the arms have to work against gravity and the extra effort required makes extra demands on the heart. So introduce these moves gradually, especially when there may be people in your class who rarely raise their hands above their heads in the course of their normal daily routine.

Relate the moves to everyday activities, such as stretching a little further than normal to reach something, making exaggerated movements when brushing the hair, getting dressed, and so on. (See Chapter 6 on Daily living activities).

Level 5 – Adding strengthening exercises

Strength training is critical if joint stability, bone and muscle strength is going to be preserved or even increased. Remember to vary the routine regularly or the muscles will get used to the same old routine. Once again, start slowly, using just the weight of the limbs and body. Extra attention must be paid to breathing rate as there is often a temptation to breath hold during the most difficult part of a move. Good posture and form is vital to ensure the moves remain safe and effective. Below are a few simple moves you can start with. Introduce these moves following a warm up period that has included a few stretches on the areas you plan to strength train. Repeat these moves 2–4 times.

Palm press (No. 9) and shoulder pull (No. 10) for chest and upper back muscles

Finger lifts (No. 22) and fingers to thumb (No. 25) for the fingers

Wrist pushover (No. 29) and wrist and grip strengthener (No. 31) for the wrist

Head press (No.12) for the neck

Rocking feet (No. 44) for calves

Leg extensions (No. 34) for thighs

Back press (No. 14) for the back

Chair push ups (No. 8) and sit to stand (No. 39) for shoulders, arms and legs.

Level 6 – Adding resistance bands to strength training

To prepare for this level, take another look at the section 'Adding resistance to exercise' (at the end of Chapter 5) and the whole of Chapter 4 'Safety first'. Then try the exercises (Nos. 50–55) without resistance bands until everyone feels comfortable with the moves, and are performing them well, with the correct breathing techniques.

Even if there is only time for one or two strengthening exercises a couple of times a week, something is better than nothing. Every day should include a little time for relaxation, deep breathing and posture review.

Making exercise fun

Most of us have taken up some kind of exercise or activity and then stopped because we simply became bored with it. For many of us, it is not enough to understand that exercise helps to keep us healthy. To remain motivated we have to enjoy doing the activity, there has to be variety and – most of all – it needs to be fun. Here are a few ideas to get you started.

Musical instruments

Create your own music to add new interests and challenges to an exercise session. A wide variety of simple musical instruments can be found in children's toyshops; they are safe, brightly coloured, easy to use and lots of fun. Look around for things like flutes, triangles, small 'bongo' drums, tambourines, castanets and 'jingle bells' on sticks. Or make your own instruments. Maracas can be easily made out of small, empty mineral water bottles. Paint the bottles in bright colours and fill them approximately a quarter full with dried beans, pasta, rice, eggshells, sand etc. These fillings add a little weight to the exercises and make interesting noises when shaken. Use the musical instruments to accompany taped music in the endurance section when the pace is a little quicker and everyone is warmed and prepared to work a little harder. Many care homes have a piano in the sitting room, there are bound to be a number of talented pianists living or working in the home, ask around for volunteers who would enjoy playing a few songs for your class. People are generally very pleased to be asked to play.

Music

The older people you work with will have lots of ideas about the kind of music they would like to exercise to and sing a long with. Show songs, popular classics, old time musical hall tunes from the thirties, forties and fifties, along with wartime favourites are always appreciated. It is much easier to choreograph exercises that make the body move safely and rhythmically if the music has a steady, strong, consistent beat. Music with a slower beat is suitable for warm up, cool down and stretching. Choose a slightly faster beat for the endurance section of the programme. Try taping a selection of music from various tapes and discs onto a blank cassette tape in the order you will need them. This allows the music to run smoothly through each segment of the exercise session, avoiding unnecessary interruptions to change tapes or discs. Always start very slowly with all segments of the class and increase the pace as individuals become comfortable and confident with the moves.

Themes

This is an opportunity to experiment and have a lot of fun with music and dance steps from different countries and cultures such as the Irish jig, French can can, West Indian calypso, American line dancing, and so on. My class members enjoy playing the maracas to a background of Latin American music to which we perform a basic salsa step (exercise No.49) and the tropicana wiggle (No. 41). To further the Latin American theme we are learning a little Spanish – just one or two words a week. We now greet and say good-bye to each other in Spanish. Try

dressing up for the part, simply done by using residents' shawls and placing fabric or paper flowers in the hair. The men are not expected to go along with the flower in the hair bit, but they do enjoy waving a shawl or other piece of cloth around in 'matador' style.

Parachutes

This is a fun, sociable group activity and a very good exercise for the hands, arms and shoulders. The cooperation of the whole class is required to keep the parachute moving rhythmically. For the parachute I use an old tablecloth or sheet. Real silk parachutes can be bought (see Resources section for suppliers), but these can be expensive. The class members sit in a circle and everyone holds firmly onto one end of the parachute. Starting with small movements, the parachute is gently shaken up and down. Gradually the movements become larger and the parachute is thrown upwards and then allowed to drop slowly downwards. Add more complicated moves, such as a 'Mexican wave', once the group has good control over the parachute.

Scarves

Brightly coloured scarves of varying weights and textures also encourage upper body movement. Many of the ladies in my groups have their own selection of scarves they are happy to use, or look through your local charity shops or jumble sales for excellent bargains. You can also make your own scarves from old pillowcases, sheets and clothing.

Beanbags

These are fun to catch and throw. Avoid making the filling too heavy or they will be difficult to throw and lethal to catch. Stitch a pocket size of brightly coloured fabric around three of the edges, fill with dried beans or rice, then stitch the remaining seam closed. Or if you wish to avoid the trouble of stitching, place the filling into a strong plastic zip lock bag and then simply place the bag inside an old clean sock. Tie the sock closed to prevent the bag from slipping out.

Chapter 8

Good mental health

The ancient Greeks believed that the mind and body were inseparably connected, that a healthy body produced a healthy mind and similarly a relaxed stress free mental state was less likely to lead to disease and suffering. Certainly it is not inevitable that we must 'lose our marbles' as we grow older. Older people can remain mentally agile given the right circumstances. Physical exercise can benefit the mind as well as the body when the moves are stimulating and challenging[1]. Good mental health also includes the ability to relax the mind and the body. This chapter looks at a few relaxation and deep breathing techniques that may have benefits for us all.

Stress

Stress has many dimensions and people will vary as to what they will find stressful. Too much or too little stress can lead to a variety of illnesses including poor sleep, irritability, despair, exhaustion, palpitations, loneliness and isolation. However, not all stress is bad and we all know individuals who seem to thrive under pressure, often producing their best performances in such conditions. In fact, without some stress we would all be bored and apathetic. Problems arise when unwanted changes (stressors) become too intense or long lasting, and we can neither fight nor flee the situation. Stress then becomes distress.

Perfect tension

To get an idea of the effects of stress we can imagine ourselves as violins playing beautiful music because our strings are perfectly tensed. If the strings become loose there is no music, just unpleasant noises. Tighten the strings too far and the tension may become so great that the strings snap.

Older people get stressed too

Why should those people in supported settings feel stressed when their every need is taken care of? No bills to pay, no shopping, cleaning, or cooking responsibilities and time to do as they please. Yet these are often precisely the reasons why they feel anxious. Older people tell me they miss the shopping, cleaning and cooking as this helped to keep them busy and made them feel useful. Even paying bills was missed by those who had always controlled their own finances. Then imagine handing over your most basic, intimate needs to someone else (usually several people) because you are not strong enough to take yourself to the bathroom.

While most residents are grateful and secure in the knowledge that professionals and other residents are always there for support through times of illness or difficulty, there are also tensions and conflicts associated with living in any kind of institutional setting. For example, residents who share a bedroom may find it difficult to get private time, or their sleep may be interrupted by noisy room mates or neighbours. There may be some residents who are difficult to get on with but walking away from a conflict is not an option if you have a mobility problem. Small annoyances accumulate so that even simple things make some people 'blow a fuse'.

This is what one care home resident had to say on the subject:

> I'm happy to a certain extent, although I do miss my peaceful cottage, it can get quite hectic here at times. I suppose it's better this way because I know I can't look after myself properly. I feel healthy but I just can't get about and I get irritated with myself and sometimes even with other people about that. It's very frustrating.

Table 8.1 The benefits of relaxation

- Blood pressure and heart rate are lowered
- Breathing rate is slowed
- Anxiety is reduced
- Relaxation concentrates the mind
- An opportunity for peace and a break from the day's tensions are created

The atmosphere in care homes is also an important issue for those working there. Tense situations may take their emotional toll when carers are giving continuously to others. Only recently a senior carer in one of the homes I visit asked if my next discussion with the residents could include, 'how to live peacefully with each other'.

However, it is not possible to take away all the stress from our own lives, or the lives of the people we care for. Stress is an inescapable part of life. But, clearly, we can have a better day and perhaps feel fewer aches and pains if we can reduce some of the unnecessary stress and tension in our lives.

Preparing for relaxation

I like to end every exercise class with a relaxation period that includes other techniques such as deep breathing and visualisation. You might also like to try these and also explore other possibilities such as meditation, yoga and T'ai Chi.

Time to relax

The relaxation period can be as long or as short as you like. It is a perfect way to finish an exercise session. I like to relax with my class for the length of a piece of music, which generally means anything from three to ten minutes. Most tapes and compact discs carry information about the length of each track. We also try to complete this period so that it coincides with the arrival of the tea trolley!

Atmosphere

Take time to think about the surroundings for this special time. Distractions can quickly spoil the atmosphere. Close sitting room doors and perhaps hang a little notice on the door to prevent unwanted interruptions. If it is possible to draw a few curtains and turn off or dim the lights, this will help to create a calm atmosphere appropriate for this period.

Soothing sounds

Participants are invited to choose the mood from a generous selection of music and quite often residents bring their own tapes. Occasionally we are treated to a live performance of 'Ave Maria' from one of the residents. Specific relaxation tapes are now available from most music outlets that include sound effects of for example, rippling water, whale sounds or singing birds. Or just look through your own music collection for the more peaceful, soothing tracks. I also adjust my voice for this calmer period, using a slower, softer tone, yet still loud enough for those with hearing difficulties.

The Mitchell method

The relaxation technique suggested in this book is based on Laura Mitchell's method of relaxation[2]. This method is used widely by our National Health Service and private practitioners all over the world. The technique shows how to recognise the differences between tension and relaxation. The method then demonstrates how to develop the skill of relaxation. I prefer to use a systematic head to toe approach to make certain no area is forgotten.

Start by inviting the class to get into a comfortable position. Make sure chairs support the neck and back, with the feet placed firmly on the floor. I use a couple of telephone books for those whose legs do not reach the floor. Hands can rest on chair arms or in the person's lap. There are no hard and fast rules about how to conduct this section of the class. The following is a typical example of the instructions I have used for the relaxation period:

- Think about relaxing, allowing the chair to support your head and back. Place your hands on the armchair rest or in your lap. Palms are facing upwards, fingers are relaxed.

- Allow your eyelids to feel heavy. Close your eyes if you wish but do not screw them up.

- Concentrate and try to put all other things out of your mind.

- Think of lifting your forehead up towards the hairline and down the back of the head. Stop when your forehead feels smooth. Feel your forehead settling down to its natural position.

- Now we work our way down to the jaw. Keeping the mouth closed, pull down the lower jaw, until the teeth are separated, then stop. Feel your tongue resting in the middle of your mouth, with the tip touching the lower teeth.

- Before we make our way down to the shoulders, think about taking the weight away from your head and neck. Your head weighs around ten pounds – a lot of weight to balance on your neck. Push the back of your head into the chair and then stop. *Never* allow the head to tip backwards, this may make you feel dizzy and can even cause neck injury. Feel the chair taking the weight of your head and the neck slightly stretching.

- The shoulders are a magnet for tension and can end up around our ears when we are stressed. Pull the shoulders down towards the feet and then stop. Feel the shoulders gently rise back to find a comfortable position away from your ears.

- With the elbows well supported on the chair arm or lap, gently and slowly push the elbows away from your side. Stop when the elbows are slightly open. Feel the elbow joints open up and the weight of the elbows taken by the supporting chair arms or lap.

- Allow this feeling to work its way down to the hands and fingers. Stretch the fingers and thumbs out so they are long and open. Then slowly bend the hands back at the wrists. Stop and allow the fingers and hands to gently fall back onto the support. Feel the fingers and thumbs make contact with the support.

- We move now to the body. Push the body into the chair and then stop. Feel fully supported by your chair.

- You will have used your legs to help push yourself back into the chair. So move the legs around now so that the feet are slightly pointing out to the sides – your knees should be facing in the same direction as the toes. Feel this new position.

- Now think about your knees. Move them so they also feel comfortable and then stop. Feel this comfortable position.

- From the knees we can continue working down towards the feet and toes. Stretch the toes, then point them down towards the floor whilst slightly raising the heels off the floor. The toes are taking the weight. Then stop and allow heels to return to the floor. Feel the feet gently settling back onto the floor so that the weight is evenly distributed throughout both feet.

Taking a mental vacation

Continue to concentrate on how comfortable your body now feels. You may wish to repeat the exercise top to toe or simply enjoy the way you now feel. Try to recall a happy memory or take a mental vacation where you imagine somewhere very pleasant, a place you may have visited in the past or would like to visit in the future. Maybe it is a cosy place in front of a roaring fire on a cold and frosty evening. Or perhaps the place is warm and bright and you can feel the sun on your face as you imagine lying on the beach or walking in the sunny countryside.

Breathing

Relaxation techniques also help to focus attention on the way we breathe. Efficient breathing helps to get rid of wastes and brings oxygen to every part of the body. Yet most of the time we breathe in a shallow way which involves mainly the upper chest area. This kind of breathing reduces the amount of oxygen we take into our lungs and also encourages the lungs, diaphragm and rib muscles to become weak and lose their elasticity. As with other muscles in our body, our chest muscles can benefit from regular exercise.

Keep at least a few minutes available for deep breathing exercises at the end of each class. This important period helps to wake up and refresh the mind and body, ready to face the remainder of the day. Once everyone becomes familiar with the breathing techniques and experiences the benefits it brings, deep breathing can also be used at other times of the day. For example, when waking up or preparing for sleep. Or as a way to deal with stress and tension, we are all familiar with the advice to 'take a deep breath' before facing difficult situations.

Once again, I use the basic principles of the Laura Mitchell[2] method of deep breathing since her techniques have been gathered specifically with older people in mind.

- These deep breathing exercises can be practised whilst lying down or sitting in a chair. Sometimes deep breathing can make you feel dizzy, therefore never practice these deep breaths whilst standing.

- Sit as tall as you can in the chair (or support the neck with a small pillow if lying down).

- Take a deep breath in through your nose. Feel the chest expand as you breath in and the ribs open outwards.

- Then slowly breathe out through your nose. Feel the chest getting smaller and the ribs falling back to their original position.

- Now allow your breathing to return to normal before trying again.

- This time, place a hand just below the ribs so you can feel the chest and stomach area rise as you breathe in and then fall as you breathe out.

- Try not to hold your breath; the breathing in and out process should be smooth and continuous.

- Take time once again to let your breathing settle before taking one more deep breath.

- Keep your hand lightly on your chest, just below the ribs. Concentrate on breathing slowly in through your nose. Feel the air entering your nose and lungs. Be aware of your chest and ribs slowly rising – then exhale slowly. Now feel the chest return to its natural position.

- As you allow your breathing to return to normal once again, think of how refreshed you now feel. Try to remember this feeling and use the deep breathing whenever you need to find a little extra peace and energy.

Table 8.2 The benefits of deep breathing

- Exercises lungs, chest muscles and diaphragm
- Regulates breathing rhythm
- Promotes relaxation
- Helps to diffuse tension and strain
- May help to ward off minor infections
- Refreshes the mind and body

References

1 Lauder, W. (1993) Health promotion in the elderly. *British Journal of Nursing*, Vol.2, No.8, pp.401–404.

2 Mitchell, L. (1988) *The Magic of Movement: A Tonic for Older People*. Age Concern, Surrey (out of print).

Chapter 9

*H*ealth forum

The health forum brings residents together into an informal discussion group where they can explore health issues and understand more about the potential benefits of exercise in their own lives. Outlining the rewards of exercise may also provide people with the knowledge, attitudes and motivation to increase activity. This type of forum can be developed from a simple question and answer session held at the end of each exercise class.

The forum is also open to anyone else who is interested in sharing their health knowledge and experiences, such as residential staff and visiting relatives. Even those residents who choose not to join the exercise sessions will often join the discussion groups. And in some cases, once the connection between exercise and health has been made, they may even decide to try the exercises.

Developing a health forum of your own

Begin by taking a few minutes, say once a month, at the end of an exercise class for reflection and discussion. This is also a good opportunity to outline future goals. Encourage lively participation with brainstorming or a question and answer discussion. For example, ask everyone to give the first word that comes into their head when you say 'physical activity'. Write these words down in large bold letters on a flip chart or large piece of paper, then use these words to explore feelings and beliefs about the subject. Choose a time of day such as tea time for an informal, non-threatening atmosphere where people feel that their ideas are appreciated and that they can respond freely without being criticised.

Develop the forum by suggesting a 10–20 minute period where a specific topic, chosen ahead of time, can be explored. People will want to join in if it is something that concerns them or it is a topic that they are really interested in. Ask class members for their ideas or think about an issue that may have been previously mentioned and make this your subject for the health forum. You could introduce the subject by saying for example something along the lines of the following:

> I know a few of you have mentioned problems with arthritis. I thought we could take a closer look at this subject when we hold our next discussion group. I will see if I can find some information on the subject and perhaps you will think about your experiences of arthritis. Even if you are fortunate enough not to suffer from the complaint, most of us will know someone who has arthritis. It would be useful to swap all we know about arthritis and perhaps learn from each other the different ways of handling this problem.

Health forum topics

At the end of this chapter you will find a few examples of subjects you might like to include in a health forum. Some of these topics may appear to be a little heavy at first, but the idea is to highlight the positive, practical points people can take when faced with health problems. Taking the subject of arthritis once more, it is quite sufficient simply to outline the two common types of arthritis:

- Osteoarthritis (wear and tear of weight bearing joints such as neck, back, hips, and knees);

- Rheumatoid arthritis (inflammation of smaller joints such as hands, fingers, wrists, ankles and feet).

The remaining time can then be spent discussing the role of exercise in arthritis, practising specific exercises, investigating available gadgets and equipment that make daily living easier and encouraging those who suffer from arthritis to set up their own support groups with other residents.

Information sources

Once the subject has been chosen, a little background search will provide an outline of the main points. It is most important to keep it simple. The information must also be reliable. Try the patient's library in your doctor's surgery. I find the books here are excellent for useful, practical information in an easy to understand format. These books are also often a source for relevant organisations, such as the Arthritis Association. For a small fee, or often for the cost of only a stamped, addressed envelope, these associations can provide further information, posters, brochures, and similar material. Photocopy and enlarge the illustrations for handouts, or make a simple copy onto a flip chart. These add visual interest, and help to get the information over. Remember that many residents may have difficulties with hearing or sight. Use large print and keep the message brief.

Communication points

No one wants to sit and be preached or lectured at. The health forum leader is a facilitator who provides the support people need to learn by setting the scene and encouraging group discussion. Being an effective facilitator of learning requires many of the qualities already used to lead an activity group, such as patience, sensitivity, creativity and the ability to appreciate that older people have a valuable contribution to make. Encourage participation with open ended questions that require more than a 'yes' or 'no' response. An appropriate open ended question might be something like, 'What is the best advice you could give to a fellow arthritis sufferer?'

The session is also more likely to be effective if the leader is positive, enthusiastic and knowledgeable. But do not be tempted to blind everyone with science, even if you know a great deal about the subject. Overwhelming people with information will alienate or bore them. You are not expected to know all the answers to all the questions. Unanswered questions simply become homework for the whole group and can be tackled again at future meetings.

Guest speakers

Specialist subjects can be handled by guest speakers. For example, the chiropodist may agree to come in and talk about common foot problems and care of the feet. Perhaps you will have to look no further than your care home to find other specialist speakers. For example, try approaching colleagues who may have additional training or knowledge in areas such as counselling, mental health, wound care, rehabilitation etc. Visitors to the home, such as relatives, district nurses, health visitors and even the local vicar may be happy to give a short talk if they are given sufficient notice. Finally, do not overlook the residents themselves who have a reservoir of experience to draw on.

One of the most successful guest speakers to visit our group was my neighbour, Kathleen (whom I have mentioned earlier). Kathleen

had recently been awarded the MBE for lifetime services to others and the residents enjoyed hearing about her big day at Buckingham Palace. They were fascinated to see her medal, photographs, and letters from the Queen. Whilst this talk was not strictly about health, it did lift spirits and demonstrate that older people are valued and respected members of society.

Table 9.1 Points for a successful forum

- Keep it simple
- Be a good listener
- Respect everyone's contribution
- Give positive reinforcement and encourage further participation, for example, 'that's an interesting point, tell us more'
- Add interest with posters, handouts, flip charts, quizzes, games, role play etc
- Emphasise positive, practical points
- Be prepared to learn from the group
- Repeat advice and important points at the end
- Accept feedback – both positive and negative

Health forum subject ideas

The following is by no means a comprehensive list of ideas, but you will find them helpful in getting you started. You can visit libraries, surgeries, colleges, newsstands etc. for further ideas and information. Most of all, ask residents what they would like to talk about. You will find that it is possible to relate activity and exercise to virtually any subject you cover – this really is the challenge and goal of a health forum.

Healthy diet

Just about everyone has something to say about food. We understand that a healthy diet is necessary for a healthy body, but it is also vital for a healthy mind. Vitamin deficiencies may contribute to memory and learning impairment[1].

Although shopping for food and cooking is no longer under the control of people who are in care – it is (and should be) possible for residents to have some level of control over their own diets. Most residential homes offer a daily menu to choose from. Use these menus to discuss healthy food choices. Accepting catering circumstances and budget constraints, care home managers and caterers may be open to requests for additional or alternative foods that support a resident's idea of a healthy diet.

Try these ideas too:

- Start the discussion by asking everyone to complete the sentence 'My favourite food is … '

- Discuss the way food is advertised on the television and in magazines.

- Ask residents for their favourite recipes.

- Collect lots of colourful food pictures from magazines to illustrate basic food groups. Then invite residents to compose ideal meals/snacks with the pictures. Stick the illustrations onto a flip chart or large piece of paper.

- Use the same illustrations to demonstrate some of the effects certain foods have on our bodies. You will need to make a few large cards with headings such as 'good for healthy bowels' and 'good for healthy skin' etc. Then invite the class to place the food pictures under each heading.

Good posture

You may be able to borrow a few charts or even a simple anatomy model (from a nursing or physiotherapy department) to demonstrate the shape of the spine.

Invite a physiotherapist to give a short talk or to supply you with basic information on the subject. The talk should include tips on sitting, lifting, bending and relaxation.

Write to the National Back Pain Association (address provided in the Resources section) for leaflets showing gentle exercises for older people. Check with the doctor that these exercises are suitable before sharing the information.

Humour

Outline the physical and mental advantages of 'a jolly good laugh' (see Chapter 2).

Make up limericks, think of alternative captions for cartoons, and swap 'doctor, doctor' jokes.

Ask residents to share their funniest life experiences. We've had lots of fun with this one. I remember when Enid, one of the residents, told us this story. She used to get plenty of exercise by cycling to work each day and, when the weather was nice, would sometimes vary her route and cycle along by the river. One summer evening, on her way home from work, she saw someone in the river who appeared to be in distress. Without regard for her own safety, Enid jumped into the river to rescue this person. As she approached the 'young lad' and reached out to help him, he suddenly stopped splashing about, turned to Enid and said 'It's all right missus – I can swim'.

Complementary therapies

There has been quite a growth in the use of complementary therapies in partnership with traditional medicine. Many care homes now have regular visits from complementary therapists such as reflexologists and aromatherapists. These practitioners may be happy to give a short talk about the work they do or provide information about their work. Once again, libraries are a good source of information, or look out for articles on this subject on popular newsstand magazines.

Aromatherapy (essential) oils can now be bought from the high street chemist. Try experimenting with a little essential lavender oil. Add a few drops of lavender to a little coconut or grapeseed oil (just two drops of lavender to a teaspoon of coconut or grapeseed oil). This mixture can then be rubbed gently onto the backs of each others hands or arms (avoid vigorous robbing of the skin, especially in those who have painful arthritic conditions). Try a few drops (3–4 drops) of the lavender oil in the bath or use just one drop on the pillow or a handkerchief for a relaxing soothing effect.

Exercise is for everyone

You will find lots of information in this book to help you with this one.

There is generally a wide variety of opinions on this subject. Use the 'round robin' approach again and start by asking each person the question, 'What is your idea of good exercise?' Make a list of all the answers on a flip chart or large piece of paper and use these as a basis for further exploration.

For example, if someone says their idea of good exercise is walking – then discuss the benefits of this activity. These may include 'good for the heart and circulation', 'builds strong bones and muscles in the legs', 'cheers you up' etc. Show how the benefits of walking can still be achieved, even when mobility is very poor, with chair exercises which can mimic the action of walking (Exercises 3 and 32).

Write to your local Health Education Authority (see resource section of this book) to ask if they can provide posters, brochures or other material specifically aimed at older people and exercise. Display these posters in the care home and help to change the belief that exercise is only for younger people.

Reference

1   Barnett R. *Is Aging Old Hat? (1991)* U.S News & World Report. Oct 7, v.111 n.15 p.A7(1).

Chapter 10

Exercise, older people and health improvement: a health promotion perspective

Piers Simey

'The wise, for cure, on exercise depend' *John Dryden*

Developing local physical activity opportunities for older people seems such clear common sense. Physical, mental and social benefits are soon visible and the best sessions generate frequent laughter, a sure sign of enjoyment. Appropriate exercise sessions are an immensely practical way to meet many of the needs of older people. But when compared to other health behaviours such as smoking and nutrition, exercise sessions are not widespread, quality is questioned and promotion is largely under funded. At a time when resources are gradually going towards meeting the needs of the most vulnerable, it is difficult to argue against the need for targeted exercise programmes focusing on older people.

This chapter aims to highlight how to gain and sustain support for community based exercise programmes targeting older people. It is written for a number of audiences who can collectively contribute to the success of an exercise initiative. It would all be so simple if we were guided to the right people, blank cheques were written and all background organisation was arranged. In reality, it is often unclear who to approach, budgets are tight and any new initiative (exercise or otherwise) must prove itself as a local priority.

An additional hurdle is that, in keeping with the rest of the population, many decision makers will themselves be inactive, associating exercise with images of lycra, sweat, and the grimaces of young faces. Balance is needed, therefore, between sensitive persuasion of the individuals approached and direct appeal to the priorities of the organisation they work for.

Partnership and alliance work will be a core theme of this chapter, as it is only through joint work that lasting changes can be achieved. Tailored exercise for older people sits well within the Government's strategy for health improvement and this central drive can be a starting point for revitalising or creating partnerships. Chair based exercise programmes can be safely applied, are effective in meeting specific practical aims and their delivery is enhanced by training; evaluation has also helped to reassure doubters. These aspects are critical for credible long-term programmes and will be covered in greater depth later.

Where does exercise fit within new public health agendas?

A number of recent policy initiatives (see Table 10.1) aim to improve the quality of life, independence, social networks and health of older people, as well as reduce their experience of health inequalities. Choosing to live a healthier lifestyle (exercising, eating well, not smoking) is secondary to tackling factors such as housing, income and the environment which make a more basic contribution to health and which are often outside our immediate control. *The Independent Inquiry into Inequalities in Health*[1] stipulates the need to improve the quality of homes in which older people live, promote their mobility and develop accessible health and social services distributed according to need. A well targeted exercise programme for older people fits well within this massive agenda, but as a core component rather than an overriding priority.

Physical activity – common sense, rarely practised

The policies are positive, exercise is strongly linked to a range of factors related to health and quality of life (see Chapter 1) and older people themselves see active living as good common sense[2]. But four out of ten people aged over 50 are totally inactive and over half of sedentary people believe that they take part in enough physical activity to keep fit[3]. Physical activity may have a strong role within the new drive for health improvement, yet can it work in practice?

The promotion of successful physical activity is complex, but achievable. Part of the answer lies with the individual, as participants in any exercise programme have a diverse range of barriers, motivators, attitudes and experiences. Another part lies in our immediate environment. The healthy exercise choice (such cycling in a city) is rarely the easiest, or indeed the safest, option. But at least every-

Table 10.1 Recent government policy initiatives

Chair based exercise fits with each of these government policies:

Our Healthier Nation has set targets to reduce coronary heart disease, mental health problems, accidents and cancer; improving the health of the worst off in society is an immediate goal. Exercise can have a direct role in meeting these four priorities, particularly by reducing the risk of a serious accidental fall.

Modernising Health and Social Services aims to settle where Health Services end and Social Services begin. Both services now have a shared responsibility for promoting the independence of older people. Regular exercise is strongly related to the ability to live independently.

Modern Local Government in Touch with the People gives local authorities the duty to promote the well-being of their communities through services which are of 'best value'. High quality exercise classes are a cost effective way to improve the well-being of older people.

The New NHS – Modern, Dependable created primary care groups and trusts (PCGs/PCTs) across the country to direct services for patients. PCGs consist of GPs, community nurses, members of the public, representatives from health authorities and social services managers. On average, PCGs cover 90,000 patients within a health authority. The value of exercise for older people makes it an attractive option when tailored to local needs, such as promoting independence and preventing falls among older people.

Better Government for Older People aims to improve the quality of life for older people through listening to their voices, improved coordination of and access to services and the development of new services based on identified need. Local authorities, working in partnership, have piloted the programme and a Network of 180 local authorities and other organisations have signed up to develop their own, appropriate Better Government for Older People programmes of action. National and local fora of older people have been established so that the voices of older people can be heard and acted upon.

Health Improvement Plans (HImPs) set local priorities for action on improving health for the coming year against which local services will be judged. They will include elements from all of the above policies and are currently guided by health authorities. Exercise programmes can achieve meaningful results for some health priorities within a year. Get your exercise project into the plan by talking to the right people and it will have massive momentum (see the section below on 'Identifying funding and support').

one can exercise in a chair. Our society also retains an ageist outlook, encouraging people to rein back their activities as they age and accept an inevitable life of decline. People in powerful positions to promote physical activity with older people may not be active themselves; research has shown that they are less likely to promote physical activity than their more active colleagues[4].

Although physical activity promotion is largely common sense, some caution is needed. Empowering older people to take control of their lives is the primary goal, but close contact with primary and secondary care medical services is required first, especially if an older person has not been active for a while. This can reduce risk and help make the experience safe and effective. In

Chapter 4, Susie Dinan points out that this is not overmedicalising the issue, because the safety margins are narrowed for the older person. Only once the necessary pre-exercise assessment has been carried out can we be sure that both the chair leader/exercise professional and the older person are in a position to make more informed choices.

What should we aim to achieve?

The focus of your exercise programme should be clarified before it is launched, so that participants and supporting organisations know just what they are getting involved in. Clear direction will improve the programme's ability to market itself and enable more effective evaluation. If you don't ask what you're aiming to achieve, someone else will, usually at an awkward moment! The best programmes have clear objectives, self monitor their progress, iron out mistakes at an early stage and prove that they effectively deliver what they set out to achieve.

To maximise the benefits identified by research, exercise must be specific to the purpose identified for the programme. As we saw in Chapter 4, older people should be aware that swimming is good for the heart, circulatory system and muscle tone, but it does not specifically improve balance. If the activity includes balance training (going to an adapted aqua aerobics session instead), then improving balance is an achievable goal.

Although people know that regular physical activity is good for you, few accurately know how much is sufficient to improve health. Government agencies have set out to raise awareness of the benefits of physical activity and ensure a consistent message[5]:

- Half an hour's moderate physical activity every day will significantly improve health. Moderate physical activities include brisk walking, dancing and gardening.

- Two periods of 15 minutes of activity in a day can be beneficial and a good way to begin.

- To be of benefit, the activity should make you feel warm and breathe more heavily than usual.

These targets are realistic for improving the health of the general population and older people in particular. But moderate physical activities will not necessarily be appropriate if we wish to specifically target conditions or problems that affect older people. Preventing falling is a good example. Falls can devastate the health and quality of life of older people, but general exercise programmes will not improve physical risk factors for falling, and may even make them worse. The exercise must be adapted to focus on training balance, strength, co-ordination and reaction times. Adapted T'ai Chi has also been shown to be beneficial[6].

Exercise must be specific to the purpose[7]:

- To improve health and modify certain risk factors for falling (such as strength), moderate physical activity is appropriate.

- To reduce injurious falls, exercise should include training in balance, strength, co-ordination and reaction times.

- To reduce fractures, exercise should include bone loading in addition to the elements outlined for reducing falls.

Chair based exercise is an excellent introduction to exercise for people with a vast range of abilities, but the seated nature of the exercise means that we can only expect limited improvements in balance. More specialised programmes are required to impact on this vital risk factor for falling. For further information, see the article by Dawn Skelton and Susie Dinan[8] in the Reference list.

Appropriate qualifications and specific 'top up' professional training will enable instructors to adapt exercise programmes both to meet the needs of people with a variety of conditions and deliver what they set out to achieve.

What works in practice?

To avoid wasted time and money, it is important to put in place either something that has worked well in practice elsewhere or something that is convincingly innovative. Effectiveness and sustainability (the future for the programme once funding runs out) are the current buzzwords and funding providers will want to see how these are addressed by what you propose. The public health drive is to focus on people who take little or no physical activity, as they have the most to gain from becoming more active. In the general population, we know that the most effective interventions for encouraging sedentary people to be more active focus on the following[9]:

- Walking as the main form of physical activity.

- Moderate physical activities in addition.

- Home-based activities as the focus.

- Frequent professional contact to boost motivation.

For the more frail older people, the promotion of moderate lifestyle physical activity alone may not always be appropriate. A recent study found that after people who fell regularly were encouraged to be more active in their lives, they actually fell more regularly[10]; this may have resulted from attempting to walk more vigorously without first improving leg strength, power and gait. The American College of Sports Medicine stipulate that for frailer older people it is better to build up strength before progressing to more dynamic activities[11]. This will reduce the risk of injury and improve performance.

Chair based exercise classes are an ideal way of introducing older people to exercise. Prior assessment can identify areas of physical need, while supervised classes give the chance to guide participants in mastering the exercise techniques which can then be repeated at home. Once strength, co-ordination, balance and gait have improved, a wider range of home based exercises can be promoted with confidence.

For many older people the social opportunity of exercise classes can be their strongest motivation. Older people who take part in research trials on the effects of tailored exercise classes on falling and physical frailty may gain confidence by seeing people of a similar physical condition performing the same exercises[12]. After session refreshments give an informal chance to socialise and air worries with the peer group, rather than with a professional who may not identify with the problem. A combination of a regular exercise class, seated or otherwise, topped up with regular moderate activities will meet the basic exercise needs of most older people.

Training in chair based exercise techniques is necessary to ensure that the classes are effectively tailored to meet people's needs, that they are safely delivered to avoid unnecessary injury or alarm, and so that instructors can deal with any emergencies that may occur (see Chapter 4). An intensive chair based training course developed for health professionals is now available nationally, administered by Leicester College (see the Resources section).

Turning dreams into reality

Begin by drawing up a 'Getting started' checklist. This should include the following:

- Clear aims and an eye for the future – see the sections above on 'What should we aim to achieve?' and 'What works in practice?'

- Finding people with the skills to deliver.

- Clarifying the nature and extent of the programme (see below).

- Securing a venue.

- Resolving how to promote the sessions (see the section on 'Marketing', below).

- Determining how to evaluate the programme.

- Identifying funding and support.

The nature and extent of the programme

Many activities will be organised for older people in your local community, in addition to the wealth of opportunities for being active in daily life. Leisure centres usually run exercise programmes for people aged over 50 which enable access to a range of activities during the day at a reduced price.

More 'traditional' activities, such as tea dances and bowls, are popular and many local authorities print directories of what is available.

Gaps are more obvious in the number of active opportunities for older, more frail individuals. Chair based exercise classes can help fill this gap and can also be a springboard to other community activities, such as aqua fit, once confidence and mobility have been boosted. We know that the numbers of older people will keep rising. In business terms, few can ignore the massive potential of this growing leisure market.

Exercises that can be carried out at home should be included in all programmes to ensure continued improvements outside the exercise class. The benefits of home based exercise are long established, both for general convenience and acceptability and, when supervised and specifically targeted, to reduce falling related injuries in older people[13]. Specialist training will be required should you wish to focus on preventing falls (see the 'Resources' section).

Choosing and securing a venue

Once you know what you aim to achieve and who you want to involve in your exercise session, you'll be able to decide where you'd like to run it. The frailest older people tend to live in supported accommodation and it will be more efficient to bring the exercise to where they live, be it in halls attached to sheltered housing or sitting rooms of retirement or nursing homes. If you decide to work where people gather regularly, such as in day centres or existing social groups, you will probably not have to worry about transport. But you will often have to fit in around existing activities, mealtimes and the ever popular bingo session! If the centres value what you offer and understand your needs, you are more likely to get practical support running and promoting these sessions.

Setting up new sessions in community venues such as church halls/religious centres, community centres or leisure centres will require transport and a more intensive marketing approach (see below). If the venue is run to meet the needs of older people, there may be flexibility about pricing. Above all, owners and managers must understand that participants will need a regular time on the same day every week. The last thing you need is to do all the hard preparation work and then be faced with disrupting the schedule because of a double booking or a sudden decision to end your hiring agreement.

Marketing

Lack of awareness about what is appropriate and available locally for older people is a major stumbling block. If you are setting up a targeted exercise programme, your priority is to let as many people as possible know about it! If you get a lot of interest, you will be in a position to persuade funders to employ you for even more sessions, be it in the community or a residential setting. The flip side is that you must always be able to deliver what you promise: too often people parachute in with amazing ideas then dash expectations when they move on or simply can't meet demand.

Promotional material must be clearly laid out and legible. Use large dark print on a light background. Think about the image and messages you wish to portray – do you have a picture of an active role model to put in your information? Test out everything you produce with older people before you go to print. Leaflets are most effective when delivered by someone face to face with a recommendation rather than pushed through a letterbox, so see if you can recruit professionals or volunteers to endorse your session and do some promotional leg work. Large, bright posters on information display boards will also help.

If you are setting up a session in the community, you will need to spread the word further. Working with local press can be very effective, as they are always interested in human interest community stories. Remember that a picture says a thousand words. A photograph of a small group or an individual (if they are willing) taking part in your exercise class smiling will say much more than you could ever achieve through written description. Speak to your health promotion unit or local authority recreation department if you need help putting together a press release.

Talking to older people about what attracts their attention and where they get their information from will point you in the right direction. While word of mouth will be the best form of publicity, you need to get people talking about what your are doing. Demonstrations and talks to large social groups will help achieve that, particularly if you can do a 'double header' with someone from a 'traditional' medical background, like a GP or physiotherapist.

The final strand is to ensure that your partners are fully recognised in any promotional material, particularly if you wish to continue being funded! In an age of cuts and complaints, positive press coverage is always appreciated.

Evaluation

Evaluation is important because it ensures that the needs of those taking part are always a prime focus. Evaluation falls into three areas: evaluation of the process will show how you've got to your current situation, who's helped, who's hindered and what you will do in future to make things work better. Evaluation of your impact can be made by logging how many sessions were held in a given period and how many people attended. Finally, evaluation of your outcomes cover what tangible difference, if any, you have made to the lives of the people involved.

Process and impact evaluation can be carried out relatively simply, as long as you are systematic in recording details (class attendance) and your thoughts (partnership difficulties) as they occur. Outcome evaluation is the most difficult to prove, but it carries the greatest weight for funders. Proving that someone has without question reduced their number of falls, increased their social networks, improved their ability to live independently or raised their confidence and mood, relies on methodical and accurate assessment. In this situation, it is important to recognise your limitations and get all available support from health promotion units, medical schools or universities. Evaluation is the key to showing that your project works and is worth funding in future years.

Identifying funding and support

'When one encounters an obstruction ... one should not strive blindly to go ahead, for this only leads to complications. Ordinarily it is best to go around an obstruction and try to overcome it along the line of least resis-tance.' So advises the ancient *Chinese Book of Changes* or *I Ching*.

Chair based exercise sessions for older people may not immediately fit within the working priorities of people who may be able to help you. Lack of funding will ruin most projects, but identifying shared interests with funders will highlight lines of least resistance. Joint funding applications have a greater chance of success, as the organisations proposing the bid will be committed to carrying out the work.

Once others share your vision, your ideas become more practical. Although canvassing support may take a long time when your sessions are ready to run, getting strong backing from a variety of people will help prevent later headaches.

Essential contact

1 Health Promotion Specialists

These include Health Authorities, Local Authorities (Environmental Health), NHS Trusts. Use the phone book to find them.

Matching professional priorities

- Working for and with the community to improve their health (community development).
- Improving the health of the worst off in society (addressing health inequalities).
- Showing what interventions are more likely to work and encouraging more effective practice in projects geared towards improving health.
- Delivering on Health Improvement Plan objectives (see above).

Health Promotion Specialists will be able to link you to potential partners, provide you with health education resources and advise you on appropriate evaluation. Although not necessarily direct sources of funding, they will know about local funding opportunities and may be prepared to use their influence to champion your cause. Many Health Promotion Units work strategically, trying to turn services from treatment into effective prevention. If they support your initiative they can provide a great guide through the maze of local agendas.

Enlisting their support will depend on your angle and their specific brief. If they focus on health promotion activities for a given area (such as a borough, electoral ward or PCG), let them know about the strength of community support behind your project. If they work on specific topics, such as older people, coronary heart disease, accident prevention, mental health or physical activity, make sure you establish the strong link between your project and their topic.

Although empowering the community to improve their health is an overriding principle of the health promotion profession, with older people there is growing recognition that some form of health assessment is required first to enable the exercise to be effectively tailored to individual needs. We know that if people stick to exercise they should gain greater control over their health. The key is to ensure that the individual's condition is known before they exercise, that they are sufficiently motivated before starting and that the exercise instructor will lead a safe and effective class.

2 Sports Development/Recreation Officers – Local Authorities

Matching professional priorities

- Providing services of best value, in terms of price, effectiveness and subsidy.
- Promoting the well-being of their community.
- Delivering on Health Improvement Plan targets (if applicable).

The extent that local authority recreation departments are involved in physical activity promotion for older people will vary considerably. Some departments focus on the management of their leisure centres and the development of sporting opportunities; others add a more direct role in physical activity delivery, often being of more practical value than health promotion departments. If they are convinced about the quality of your project, they may be able to open doors to other council departments, such as social services. They will also be able to work directly with leisure centres, should you wish to make use of facilities such as swimming pools or want information on exercise programmes already available for older people.

3 Physiotherapists and occupational therapists

Matching professional priorities

- Promoting independence and quality of life.
- Rehabilitating individuals after an injury or illness.

Traditional therapy services will appreciate a trusted community based exercise opportunity to which they can refer appropriate clients. Exercise instructors will be able to gain this trust by using their skills and professionalism. The involvement of physiotherapists and occupational therapists, however minimal, in an exercise programme for older people shares skills and makes exercise assessment that much more effective.

Two-way referral may become an option, depending on the change in functional ability of the older person. For those leading chair based exercise sessions, this translates to always referring individuals for therapy if they have deteriorated significantly in condition or general health. Physiotherapists are a vital part of the exercise continuum as they will develop close therapeutic relationships with older people. Once function has improved, they will be looking to refer older people to appropriate community based services. A well led, chair based exercise class could be an ideal option for referral.

Rehabilitation principles often enhance and guide exercise practice. Advice should always be sought from physiotherapists when working with people with disabilities or those with chronic conditions, and their involvement in training exercise practitioners for this work will be invaluable.

Physiotherapy assistants are ideally placed to lead chair work as they have direct access to patients and can begin the process of associating exercise with fun more than pain. Their direct supervision by a physiotherapist enhances their appropriateness to lead chair based exercise classes.

4 Managers of facilities for older people

These would include wardens of sheltered housing complexes, day centre managers and residential home managers, for example.

Professional interests

- Offering a range of activities for residents.
- Balancing budgets.
- Promoting independence and health.

Unless you actually work for such an organisation, or know individuals who do, it is worthwhile arranging to meet such managers following contact with health promotion specialists.

It is important that your session is fully valued and supported. If you are lucky, not only will they be able to provide the venue for your class and the people to take part, but they may pay your session fees as well. Staff can assist the smooth running of the class and help organise the post class social opportunity. They can also promote the session to other people who may not initially be keen to take part, but make sure their promotional messages are accurate.

Managers may fund places on chair based exercise courses and allow their staff to attend training during working time. Once trained staff begin to lead classes at their centre, positive feedback from participants and media coverage can help reinforce this decision to invest in training.

5 Commissioners of services

Health and Local Authority managers are responsible for commissioning services.

Matching professional priorities

> ■ Promoting the independence of older people.
> ■ Putting policies into practice through effective programmes, linking with a variety of community groups and agencies.
> ■ Evaluating progress to ensure continued effectiveness.
> ■ Achieving sustainability.

Commissioners may fund chair based exercise programmes which are clearly designed to meet major local health improvement priorities. They will often oversee or be aware of a number of funding opportunities, but competition for funding is tight and you may have to rely on other agencies to appreciate and champion your programme before you contact them.

6 Primary Care Groups (PCGs)

This category includes GP practices and health centres.

Matching professional priorities

> ■ Improving the health and addressing health inequalities of their community.
> ■ Developing primary care and community services focusing on the needs of their community.
> ■ Commissioning a range of hospital services which meet their patients' needs
> ■ Implementing local Health Improvement Plans (HImPs)

If you intend to run a programme which is open for patients from a small number of GP practices, it will be worth working directly with the practices concerned. If however, your project is opened across the community, PCG approval may be required for the nature and scope of your project. There may be concern over the additional time demands and principle of doing a health check prior to exercise. Identifying GPs who are sympathetic to your ideas will be crucial, but remember that your ability to deliver the sessions effectively and safely may well be scrutinised.

Exercise referral

Most areas will have an established scheme which allows people to be referred by primary care for exercise at a local leisure centre or similar venue. The Department of Health has published quality guidelines for exercise referral schemes and there is no reason why they can not be adapted to focus specifically on older people as well as the general population.

7 Help on the ground

This includes the voluntary services and older people themselves.

Exercise opportunities span many professional and voluntary interests. The extent of local interest will differ, but there will always be groups crying out for safe effective exercise opportunities to improve the wellbeing of their members. Tapping into assistance – be it for providing clients, transport, venues or promotional support – will depend on the focus of your programme. Contact with local Age Concern groups and organisations can be a great first place to begin.

Older people themselves are the most powerful marketing resource available to you. Their interest in your programme is crucial to its future and they can help spread the word. Older people should be involved in the development, recruitment, evaluation and delivery of your programme wherever possible. They may also help by organising some of the social aspects, befriending would-be participants and those who are ill, or even by being trained to supervise exercise sessions.

Working in practice

This ground breaking initiative shows how well a co-ordinated programme of chair based exercise can work in practice. Driven by East Kent Health Promotion Service, in collaboration with the Royal Free and University College Hospital, a specific chair based exercise training course was developed in response to a local need. Physiotherapy assistants and health care assistants committed themselves to leading chair based exercise classes following intensive training over four days. A number of leaders have been trained here and across the country leading to many new chair based exercise sessions for older people.

A key factor in the programme's success has been the support available for the newly trained chair exercise leaders, both in turning the training into practical exercise sessions and in keeping newly learnt skills refreshed and up to date. Managers, tutors and health promotion staff with exercise expertise have worked closely to ensure that classes have continued as part of the everyday routine. This example of joint working has achieved national recognition and the training module has been developed nationally by Merton, Sutton and Wandsworth Health Authority and Leicester College.

Conclusion

Barriers to setting up successful chair based exercise sessions may be thrown in your path, but if you plan thoroughly and find out who your key allies are, frustration should be kept to a minimum. Exercise does not have to be imposed and most older people readily see its value. If they have informed choice and ready access to your exercise session, you will rarely lack for participants.

We are on the verge of an explosion in exercise opportunities for older people. The climate is right for working together to meet their needs and research has shown the huge potential for exercise in practice. But we must take care not to let the bubble burst. Support from primary and secondary care will help empower the older person to have a safer, more enjoyable experience of exercise. Our responsibility is to deliver high quality, accessible exercise classes across the community and actively promote them. Once this happens, we will have played our part in making an active and fitter older life more the expectation than the exception.

References

1. Acheson, D. (1998) *Independent Inquiry into Inequalities in Health*. HMSO, London.

2. Health Education Authority (1997) *Physical Activity 'At Our Age'. Qualitative Research among People over the Age of 50*. HEA, London.

3. Skelton, D.A., Young, A., Walker, A. and Hoinville, E. (1999) *Physical Activity in Later Life*. HEA, London

4. McKenna, J., Naylor, P.J. and McDowell, N. (1998) Barriers to physical activity promotion for General Practitioners and Practice Nurses. *British Journal of Sports Medicine*. 32(3): 242–247.

5. Simey, P. (1998) *Promoting Physical Activity with Carers*. HEA, London.

6. Province, M.A., Hadley, E.C., Hornbrook, M.C., Lipsitz, L.A., Miller, J.P., Mulrow, C.D., Ory, M.G., Sattin, R.W., Tinetti, M.E., Wolf, S.L. (1995) The effects of exercise on falls in elderly patients. A pre-planned meta-analysis of the FICSIT trials. *Journal of the American Medical Association*, Vol. 273, No.17, pp. 1341–1347.

7. Simey, P. and Pennington, B. (1999) *Physical Activity and the Prevention and Management of Falls and Accidents Among Older People*. HEA, London.

8. Skelton, D.A. and Dinan, S.M. (1999) Exercise for falls management: rationale for an exercise programme aimed at reducing postural instability. *Physiotherapy Theory & Practice*, Vol. 15, pp. 105–120.

9. Hillsdon, M. and Thorogood, M. (1996) A systematic review of physical activity promotion strategies. *British Journal of Sports Medicine*. Vol. 30, pp. 84–89.

10. Ebrahim, S., Thompson, P.W., Baskaran, V. and Evans, K. (1997) Randomised placebo-controlled trial of brisk walking in the prevention of post menopausal osteoporosis. *Age & Ageing*, Vol. 26, pp. 253–260.

11. ACSM (1998) Exercise and older people. *Medicine & Science in Sports & Exercise*. Vol. 30, No. 6, pp. 992–1008.

12. Personal communication with D Skelton.

13. Campbell, A.J., Robertson, M.C., Gardner, M.M., Norton, R.N., Tilyard, M.W., Buchner, D.M. (1998) Randomised controlled trial of a general practice programme of home based exercise to prevent falls in elderly women. *British Medical Journal*, Vol. 315, pp. 1065–1069.

Resources

Further reading

Sayce, V. (1999) *Exercise Beats Arthritis: An easy to follow programme of exercises*. Thorsons, HarperCollins. London.

Dinan, S and Sharpe, C. (1996) *Fitness For Life*. Piatkus, London. Available from the Exercise Association Ltd, Unit 4, Angel Gate, City Road, London EC1V 2PT.

Physical Activity Guidelines for Special Conditions (free brochure) Available from The Exercise Health Research and Development Group, Loughborough University, Ashby Road, Loughborough, Leicestershire LE11 3TU.

Mitchell, L. (1988) *The Magic of Movement: A Tonic for Older People*. Age Concern, Surrey. Currently out of print but may be available at libraries.

Teacher training

Courses are available for those who wish to train as exercise instructors to older and less able people. These qualifications also allow you to set up your own classes elsewhere in the community. Please do send a large sae when making enquiries to these organisations.

East Midlands and Pennine Training
Leicester College
Abbey Park Campus
Painters Street
Leicester LE1 3WA
E-mail: hkeighley@leicestercollege.ac.uk

EXTEND
22 Maltings Drive
Wheathampstead
Hertfordshire AL4 8QJ
Tel/Fax 01582 832 760
Web site http://gifford.co.uk/~atol/extend/

EXCEL 2000
1A North Street
Sheringham
Norfolk NR26 8LW

Tel 01263 825 670
Fax 01263 825 870

Central YMCA
Training and Development Department
112 Great Russell Street
London WC1B 3NQ
Tel 020 7343 1850

Equipment and suppliers

Crown World Marketing Ltd
Drum Grange
Nightingale's Lane
Chalfont St. Giles
Buckinghamshire HP8 4SL
Tel 01494 764 802

Suppliers of resistive fitness bands

ROMPA
Goyt Side Road
Chesterfield
Derbyshire S40 2PH
Tel 01246 211777
Fax 01246 221802
E-mail 100443.3135@compuserve.com

This catalogue includes products to increase the fun and challenge of the activity sessions, such as music tapes and CDs, musical instruments, catch balls and parachutes, as mentioned in Chapter 5

Homecraft – Chester-Care
Sidings Road
Lowmoor Road Industrial Estate
Kirby-in-Ashfield
Nottinghamshire
NG17 7JZ
Tel 01623 757955
Fax 01623 755585

This catalogue includes a wide choice of products that may help those with restricted mobility in their everyday activities

Instructional videos and cassettes

Chairbased Activities with Music by The Disabled Living Foundation
Barbara Norice
1 Irving Road
Norwich
Norfolk NR4 6RA
Tel 01603 451868

A set of three cassettes with notes describing activities with music for people who have learning and physical difficulties

'Exercise in a Chair': Top to Toe Exercise While Seated by M. Preston
Speechmark Publishing
Telford Road
Bicester
Oxfordshire OX6 OTS
Tel 01869 244644

Video demonstrating chair and supported standing exercises for older people or those who wish to instruct (formerly Winslow Press)

Fit is Fun by Excel 2000
1A North Street
Sheringham
Norfolk NR26 8LW
Tel 01263 825670
Fax 01263 825870

Exercise video for older people or those with physical difficulties

Forever Fit: Chair Exercise for the Physically Disabled and Living Longer Population by Forever Fit (USA)
Speechmark Publishing
Telford Road
Bicester
Oxfordshire OX6 OTS
Tel 01869 244733

A chair based exercise programme video for people with physical difficulties and older people

Harmonise with Exercise
Excel 2000
Available from Excel 2000, address above.

Audio cassette of simple, chair based movements and good posture tips

Other agencies and organisations

These agencies offer support for those who wish to know more about promoting physical activity for older people and those with physical difficulties. An sae would be appreciated if you write for information.

Age Concern England
Astral House
1268 London Road
London SW16 4ER
Tel 020 8765 7200
Fax 020 8765 7211

Contact the Age Concern Information Line/Factsheets Subscription for information on various factsheets and guides on 0800 00 99 66.

Alzheimer's Society
Gordon House
10 Greencoat Place
London SW1P 1PH
Tel 020 7306 0606
Fax 020 7306 0808
Website http://www.vois.org.uk.alzheimers

This national organisation has nearly 300 branches and support groups.

Arthritis Care
18 Stephenson Way
London NW1 2HD
Tel 020 7916 1500
Freephone helpline 0808 800 4050 (Mon–Fri 12noon–4pm)

Provides information, counselling, training, fund and social contact. The first port of call for anyone with arthritis. There are many smaller organisations for particular type of arthritis. Arthritis Care's helpline can provide details.

Arthritis and Rheumatism Council (for research in Great Britain and the Commonwealth)
Copeman House
St Mary's Court
St Mary's Gate
Chesterfield
Derbyshire S41 7TD
Tel 01246 558 033
Fax 01246 558 007

Publishes a news magazine in addition to other publications with the aim of helping to promote a better understanding of rheumatic diseases.

Diabetes UK
10 Queen Anne Street
London W1M OBD
Tel 020 7323 1531
Careline 020 7636 6112
Website:http//www.diabetes.org.uk

Provides help and support to people diagnosed with diabetes, their families and those who care for them.

British Geriatrics Society
31 St Johns Square
London E1M 4DN
Tel 020 7608 1369
Fax 020 7608 1041

Centre for Policy on Ageing
19–23 Ironmonger Row
London EC1V 3QP
Tel 020 7253 1787
Fax 020 7490 4206

Disabled Living Foundation
380–384 Harrow Road
London W9 2HU
Tel 020 7289 6111
Fax 020 7266 2922
Website http://www.dlf.org.uk

This organisation offers information about products that make daily living easier for those with disabilities.

Health Development Agency
(formerly the Health Education Authority)
Trevelyan House
30 Great Peter Street
London SW1P 2HW
Tel 020 7222 5300
Website http//www.active.org.uk and www.hda-online-org.uk

In 1996 the HEA launched a three year 'Active for Life' campaign to encourage more adults to exercise more often. This programme continues to develop national initiatives and support the work of local professionals. Contact its 'Active for Life' hotline on 020 7413 2637 or write to your local HEA(HDA) to find out more about this campaign and the supporting brochures, videos, posters etc. some of which are available free.

National Back Pain Association
16 Elmtree Road
Teddington
Middlesex TW11 8ST
Tel 020 8977 5474
Fax 020 8943 5318

National Osteoporosis Society
PO Box 10
Radstock
Bath BA3 3YB
Tel 01761 471771
Fax 01761 471104
Helpline 01761 472721
Website http://www.nos.org.uk

Research into Ageing
Baird House
15/17 Cross Street
London EC1N 8UW
Tel 020 7404 6878
Fax 020 7404 6816

World Health Organisation Ageing and Health Programme
WHO
Av. Appia 20
CH-1211 Geneva 27
Tel +41 22 791 3405
Fax +41 22 791 4839

E-mail: activeageing@who.ch

The United Nations launched an International Year of Older Persons on October 1st 1999. The World Health Organisation (WHO) supported this initiative by promoting the 'Global Movement for Active Ageing'.

For an address from the UN please look under http://www.un.org, then go to social action and you will find information about the initiative there.

Further information can be obtained from:

HelpAge International, London, www.oneworld.org/helpage

Fitness Professionals
113 London Road
London E13 0DA
Tel: 0990 133 434
E-mail:admin@fitpro.com

Registered exercise and fitness teachers in this organisation can buy various levels of insurance coverage. Members also receive the official magazine.

Afterword

Understanding how physical activity can maintain or improve quality of life will help us to prepare for our own old age and provide the opportunity to motivate others so that they too can age with grace and dignity. Appreciating the positive influence of exercise may also help to get rid of the many negative assumptions of what old age will be like.

The most important message must be that older people have the most to gain from regular exercise and the most to lose from inactivity[1]. I hope this book has provided the practical help you may have been searching for in order to help older people make these positive changes.

Reference

1   Fiatarone, M.A., O'Brien, K. and Rich, B.S.E. (1996) Exercise Rx for a healthier old age. *Patient Care*, October 15, pp. 145–147.

About Age Concern

Alive and Kicking is one of a wide range of publications produced by Age Concern England, the National Council on Ageing. Age Concern works on behalf of all older people and believes later life should be fulfilling and enjoyable. For too many this is impossible. As the leading charitable movement in the UK concerned with ageing and older people, Age Concern finds effective ways to change that situation.

Where possible, we enable older people to solve problems themselves, providing as much or as little support as they need. A network of local Age Concerns, supported by 250,000 volunteers, provides community-based services such as lunch clubs, day centres and home visiting.

Nationally, we take a lead role in campaigning, parliamentary work, policy analysis, research, specialist information and advice provision, and publishing. Innovative programmes promote healthier lifestyles and provide older people with opportunities to give the experience of a lifetime back to their communities.

Age Concern is dependent on donations, covenants and legacies.

Age Concern England
1268 London Road
London SW16 4ER
Tel 020 8765 7200
Fax 020 8765 7211

Age Concern Scotland
113 Rose Street
Edinburgh EH2 3DT
Tel 0131 220 3345
Fax 0131 220 2779

Age Concern Cymru
4th Floor
1 Cathedral Road
Cardiff CF1 9SD
Tel 029 2037 1566
Fax 029 2039 9562

Age Concern Northern Ireland
3 Lower Crescent
Belfast BT7 1NR
Tel 028 9024 5729
Fax 028 9023 5497

Publications from Age Concern Books

Age Concern publishes a wide variety of books for professionals working with older people.

Age Concern Training Packs

Age Concern Training Packs are ideal teaching tools for all care staff involved in the training and support of other staff. They enable trainers to effectively guide and reinforce skills and development by providing all the material necessary to run successful group training sessions.

The Training Packs:

- Can be used either as an integrated or topic-led course.

- Can be used again and again.

- Can be used by inexperienced trainers.

- Save time and money.

All contain key point overhead transparencies, aims and objectives, teaching plans, group activities and support material and handouts.

Trained Nurse's Teaching Packs: For use in the workplace to educate nursing auxiliaries, health care assistants and social services care staff

Gill Early and Sarah Miller

Concentrating on key nursing areas, these packs are designed to build on the existing knowledge and skills of untrained or unqualified staff and improve standards of care. Both packs will help to develop a better understanding of optimum client care and an improvement in practical nursing skills. They contain key point overhead transparencies, aims and objectives and teaching plans together with recommended time-scales.

Volume 1

Topics covered:

- Stomas

- Communication

- Pressure sores

- Catheters

- Physical care of the dying

- Psychological care of the dying

£27.99   0-86242-213-2

Volume 2

Topics covered:

- Promotion of continence

- Leg ulcers and wound care

- Constipation, strokes, diabetes and nutrition

£35.00   0-86242-286-8

The Successful Activity Co-ordinator's Pack: Making the best use of resources to provide activities and leisure opportunities to older people in care homes

Rosemary Hurtley and Jennifer Wenborn

This pack is aimed directly at anyone with a responsibility for providing activity and leisure opportunities for older people within residential and nursing care home settings. Full of tried and tested ideas and handby tips, it examines:

- The philosophy of 'good' health in older age.

- Work, self care and leisure.

- The role of the activity co-ordinator.

- Designing innovative programmes.

- Group-work skills.

- Effective communication – making it happen.

- Using resources effectively.

Together with sections on arts and crafts, physical activities, reminiscence work, working with people with dementia and sensory impairment, this pack is a mine of information and ideas and a key resource for anyone working in this area.

£25.00   0-86242-265-5

Nutritional Care for Older People: A handbook

June Copeman

Packed full of practical information and guidance, this book is designed to be used by all care staff concerned with food and nutrition and older people. Drawing on the latest scientific knowledge, national guidelines and accepted practice, this book will help staff develop and maintain the very best standards in all aspects of food management. Topics covered include:

■ Food environment and presentation.

■ A–Z checklist of risk factors.

■ Frequency of meals and fluid intake.

■ Stimulating a small appetite.

■ Food and mental health issues.

■ Cultural and religious issues.

■ Menu planning and recipes.

■ Nutritional needs of people with specific illnesses.

Written by an experienced nutritionist, this book stresses throughout the importance of good nutrition to health. Staff involved in food planning and management in care homes, day centres and other community settings will find this book a vital source of guidance and support.

£14.99   0-86242-284-1

Caring for Ethnic Minority Elders: A guide

Yasmin Alibhai-Brown

Addressing the delivery of care to older people from ethnic minority groups, this book highlights the impact of varying cultural traditions and stresses their significance in the design of individual care packages. The author looks at the broader framework of how elders receive care and then considers the requirements and experiences of distinct ethnic minority groups.

Designed to help those planning the delivery of services and those working with ethnic minority elders, this book provides key guidance on developing and maintaining the highest standards in good practice and care.

£14.99   0-86242-188-8

If you would like to order any of these titles, please write to the address below, enclosing a cheque or money order for the appropriate amount (plus £1.95 p&p) made payable to Age Concern England. Credit card orders may be made on 0870 44 22 044 (individuals) or 0870 44 22 120 (AC federation, other organisations and institutions). Fax: 01626 323318.

Age Concern Books
PO Box 232
Newton Abbot
Devon TQ12 4XQ

Age Concern Information Line/Factsheets subscription

Age Concern produces 44 comprehensive factsheets designed to answer many of the questions older people (or those advising them) may have. These include money and benefits, health, community care, leisure and education, and housing. For up to five free factsheets, telephone: 0800 00 99 66 (7am–7pm, seven days a week, every day of the year). Alternatively you may prefer to write to Age Concern, FREEPOST (SWB 30375), ASHBURTON, Devon TQ13 7ZZ.

For professionals working with older people, the factsheets are available on an annual subscription service, which includes updates throughout the year. For further details and costs of the subscription, please write to Age Concern at the above Freepost address.

Index